Cancer Treatment and Research

Volume 184

Series Editor

Steven T. Rosen, Duarte, CA, USA

This book series provides detailed updates on the state of the art in the treatment of different forms of cancer and also covers a wide spectrum of topics of current research interest. Clinicians will benefit from expert analysis of both standard treatment options and the latest therapeutic innovations and from provision of clear guidance on the management of clinical challenges in daily practice. The research-oriented volumes focus on aspects ranging from advances in basic science through to new treatment tools and evaluation of treatment safety and efficacy. Each volume is edited and authored by leading authorities in the topic under consideration. In providing cutting-edge information on cancer treatment and research, the series will appeal to a wide and interdisciplinary readership. The series is listed in PubMed/Index Medicus.

Charles Bennett • Courtney Lubaczewski •
Bartlett Witherspoon

Editors

Cancer Drug Safety and Public Health Policy

A Changing Landscape

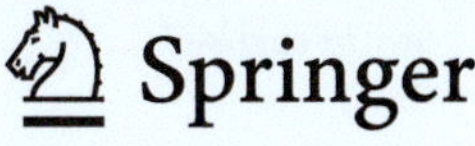
Springer

Editors
Charles Bennett
College of Pharmacy
University of South Carolina
Columbia, SC, USA

Courtney Lubaczewski
College of Pharmacy
University of South Carolina
Columbia, SC, USA

Bartlett Witherspoon
College of Pharmacy
University of South Carolina
Columbia, SC, USA

ISSN 0927-3042	ISSN 2509-8497	(electronic)
Cancer Treatment and Research
ISBN 978-3-031-04404-5	ISBN 978-3-031-04402-1	(eBook)
https://doi.org/10.1007/978-3-031-04402-1

This Springer imprint is published by the registered company Springer Nature Switzerland AG
The registered company address is: Gewerbestrasse 11, 6330 Cham, Switzerland

Preface

Policy is a critical area of research in the field of oncology. Understanding the factors that determine the quality of care is important for providing comprehensive treatment.

Serious adverse events associated with antibiotics, the topic of the chapter by Champigneulle, Bennett, Bennett, and Martin, threaten the health of patients and limit their quality of life. On the other hand, copies of patented biologicals called biosimilars, discussed by Nagai, Witherspoon, and Bennett, exist as an alternative treatment option for cancer patients. Both of these chapters assess the cost and benefits of commonly utilized treatment options in order to ensure the best patient outcome.

It is important that the information provided about these drugs is the most accurate. Chen, Yang, and Bennett describe how better transparency is needed in disseminating safety information to providers and patients. Citizen petitions are a way to report recorded safety data. Possible action suggested in these petitions described by Martin, Ray, and Bennett include label changes or boxed warnings. As illustrated by Taylor and colleagues, there are concerns in safe reporting of these adverse events. Lawsuits and fear of jeopardizing existing collaborations could make clinicians hesitant to share their findings.

There are correlations between drugs and adverse reactions that are documented by clinicians. One of these reactions noted by Bennett, Witherspoon, and Carson is nephrogenic fibrosis following treatment with GBCAs. This disease limits the quality of life so it is important to consider if taking the medication is worth the risk. Different adverse drug reactions can occur with different medications such as the link between rituximab and leukoencephalopathy discussed by Bennett, Witherspoon, and Carson. This clinical and epidemiologic data is essential for providers to receive so they can make decisions in the best interest of their patient's safety.

There is a various methodology that can be used to compile this safety data. As described by Yarnold and colleagues, these methods include logistic regression with an independent variable, attributes with identical level of influence, and equivalent coefficients. Another way to investigate adverse drug data is the ANTICIPATE methodology presented by Bennett, Schooley, and Hoque. This facilitates systemic analysis of four sADRs among chronic kidney disease patients.

Important components of this method include signal detection, cost analyses, and toxicity eradication recommendations. Reporting through these methods can lead to consequences by clinicians. These are described by Lubaczewski and colleagues to include loss of clinician jobs and costly legal settlements. These findings highlight the importance of Data Safety Monitoring Boards and anonymous reporting to encourage clinicians to report all findings imperative to patient well-being. Alternative adverse event reporting platforms including vaccine databases and social media are highlighted by Bennett and Champigneulle. Additionally, the relevance of utilizing genetic markers to identify at-risk patients is described by A. Bennett. In sum, these twelve chapters in this edition highlight some important parts of oncology drug reactions and their reporting. We are pleased to have had the opportunity to edit this work.

<table>
<tr><td>Columbia, USA</td><td>Charles Bennett, M.D., Ph.D.</td></tr>
<tr><td></td><td>Courtney Lubaczewski</td></tr>
<tr><td></td><td>Bartlett Witherspoon, MBA</td></tr>
</table>

Contents

Editors and Contributors

About the Editors

Charles Bennett, M.D. Ph.D. MPP SmartState Chair and Frank P. and Josie M. Fletcher Chair of Medication Safety and Efficacy and Director, SmartState Center for Medication Safety and Efficacy, is also a Visiting Scholar at the City of Hope National Cancer Institute Designated Comprehensive Cancer Center in Duarte, California and is the co-editor of this book, Cancer Policy (2nd Edition). Dr. Bennett is a Phi Beta Kappa and High Honors graduate in mathematics from Swarthmore College, earned his medical degree in 1981 from the University of Pennsylvania Perelman School of Medicine, and completed internal medicine, hematology, and oncology training at the Michael Reese Hospital and the University of Chicago Pritzger School of Medicine before completing his Ph.D. and Masters In Public Policy degrees with honors in social science at the RAND Pardee Graduate School of Public Policy in Santa Monica, California. He has led a 20-year National Institutes of Health funded pharmacovigilance called the Research on Adverse Drug events And Reports (RADAR) and subsequently called to Southern Network on Adverse drug Reactions (SONAR) at the University of South Carolina College of Pharmacy.

Courtney Lubaczewski is a fourth-year undergraduate at the University of South Carolina Honors College and the co-editor of Cancer Policy with Charles Bennett M.D. Ph.D. MPP. She was a co-author on the 2021 PLOS One article on harms to physicians who report serious adverse drug reactions.

Bartlett Witherspoon, MBA is a third-year medical student at the Medical University of South Carolina and a graduate of Vanderbilt University's Master's in Business Administration program. He is an active co-investigator with Dr. Bennett and the SONAR project and has been a lead co-investigator on published manuscripts on fluoroquinolone-associated disability and on biosimilar oncology products.

Contributors

Bennett Andrew SONAR (Southern Network on Adverse Reactions) Program, University of South Carolina College of Pharmacy, Columbia, SC, USA

Bennett Charles L. SONAR (Southern Network on Adverse Reactions) Program, University of South Carolina College of Pharmacy, Columbia, SC, USA; SONAR (Southern Network on Adverse Reactions) Program, University of South Carolina Colleges of Pharmacy and Engineering, Columbia, SC, USA

Bove Cecilia York College of Pennsylvania, York, PA, USA

Carson Kenneth R. SONAR (Southern Network on Adverse Reactions) Program, University of South Carolina College of Pharmacy, Columbia, SC, USA

Champigneulle Oscar SONAR (Southern Network on Adverse Reactions) Program, University of South Carolina College of Pharmacy, Columbia, SC, USA

Chen Brian SONAR (Southern Network on Adverse Reactions) Program, University of South Carolina College of Pharmacy, Columbia, SC, USA

Godwin Ashley C. SONAR (Southern Network on Adverse Reactions) Program, University of South Carolina Colleges of Pharmacy and Engineering, Columbia, SC, USA

Hoque Shamia SONAR (Southern Network on Adverse Reactions) Program, University of South Carolina College of Pharmacy, Columbia, SC, USA; SONAR (Southern Network on Adverse Reactions) Program, University of South Carolina Colleges of Pharmacy and Engineering, Columbia, SC, USA

Hrushesky William R. SONAR (Southern Network on Adverse Reactions) Program, University of South Carolina College of Pharmacy, Columbia, SC, USA

Knopf Kevin SONAR (Southern Network on Adverse Reactions) Program, University of South Carolina College of Pharmacy, Columbia, SC, USA

Lubaczewski Courtney R. SONAR (Southern Network on Adverse Reactions) Program, University of South Carolina College of Pharmacy, Columbia, SC, USA

Nabhan Chadi SONAR (Southern Network on Adverse Reactions) Program, University of South Carolina College of Pharmacy, Columbia, SC, USA

Nagai Sumimasa SONAR (Southern Network on Adverse Reactions) Program, University of South Carolina College of Pharmacy, Columbia, SC, USA

Olivieri Nancy F. SONAR (Southern Network on Adverse Reactions) Program, University of South Carolina College of Pharmacy, Columbia, SC, USA

Ray Paul SONAR (Southern Network on Adverse Reactions) Program, University of South Carolina College of Pharmacy, Columbia, SC, USA

Taylor Matthew SONAR (Southern Network on Adverse Reactions) Program, University of South Carolina College of Pharmacy, Columbia, SC, USA

Taylor Matthew A. SONAR (Southern Network on Adverse Reactions) Program, University of South Carolina Colleges of Pharmacy and Engineering, Columbia, SC, USA

Thomsen Henrik S. SONAR (Southern Network on Adverse Reactions) Program, University of South Carolina College of Pharmacy, Columbia, SC, USA

Ugarte Shannon SONAR (Southern Network on Adverse Reactions) Program, University of South Carolina College of Pharmacy, Columbia, SC, USA

Witherspoon Bartlett SONAR (Southern Network on Adverse Reactions) Program, University of South Carolina College of Pharmacy, Columbia, SC, USA

Yang Tony SONAR (Southern Network on Adverse Reactions) Program, University of South Carolina College of Pharmacy, Columbia, SC, USA

Yarnold Paul SONAR (Southern Network on Adverse Reactions) Program, University of South Carolina College of Pharmacy, Columbia, SC, USA

Fluoroquinolone-Associated Disability and Other Fluoroquinolone-Associated Serious Adverse Events: Unexpected Toxicities Have Emerged in Recent Years

Charles L. Bennett, Oscar Champigneulle, Andrew Bennett, Bartlett Witherspoon, and Cecilia Bove

1.1 Introduction

This study describes cases of individuals who report adverse events following consumption of the most commonly prescribed fluoroquinolone (FQ) antibiotics: ciprofloxacin, levofloxacin, or moxifloxacin. FQ antibiotics are some of the most widely prescribed antibiotics in the world. Although these antibiotics have been on the market for more than 20 years, a wide range of serious FQ-associated adverse events first became apparent in 2006 and continued to be recognized for the next 15 years.

In the United States, FQs are approved by the Food and Drug Administration (FDA) for nosocomial pneumonia, community-acquired pneumonia, complicated and uncomplicated skin and skin structure infections, chronic bacterial prostatitis, post-exposure inhalational anthrax, plague, complicated and uncomplicated urinary tract infections, acute pyelonephritis, acute bacterial exacerbation of chronic bronchitis, and acute bacterial sinusitis. Since 2015, FQs have been designated as therapeutic options only when other antibiotics are not expected to work.

C. L. Bennett · O. Champigneulle · A. Bennett · B. Witherspoon
SONAR (Southern Network on Adverse Reactions) Program,
University of South Carolina College of Pharmacy, Columbia, SC 29208, USA
e-mail: bennettc@cop.sc.edu

O. Champigneulle
e-mail: Oscar_champigneulle@brown.edu

A. Bennett
e-mail: andrew.bennett@pharm.ox.ac.uk

C. Bove (✉)
York College of Pennsylvania, York, PA 17403, USA
e-mail: cb068@bucknell.edu

© The Author(s), under exclusive license to Springer Nature Switzerland AG 2022
C. Bennett et al. (eds.), *Cancer Drug Safety and Public Health Policy*,
Cancer Treatment and Research 184, https://doi.org/10.1007/978-3-031-04402-1_1

FQ antibiotics contain Boxed Warnings for a number of issues, including the warning that FQs "have been associated with disabling and potentially irreversible serious adverse reactions that have occurred together," including tendinitis and tendon rupture, peripheral neuropathy, and central nervous system effects, which includes psychiatric reactions. In 2015, the FDA defined Fluoroquinolone-Associated Disability (FQAD) as a constellation of FQ adverse events which result in "substantial disruption of a person's ability to conduct normal life functions" and having "adverse events reported from two or more of the following body systems: musculoskeletal, neuropsychiatric, peripheral nervous system, senses (vision, hearing, etc.), skin, cardiovascular."

Individuals who experience significant FQ-related adverse drug reactions (ADRs) refer to themselves as being "floxed". A global online "floxed community" has developed over the past decade. Thousands of "floxed" individuals communicate with each other via several social media websites, including numerous Facebook groups.

Herein, we review FQ ADRs reported to the FDA, published studies, regulatory responses to questions regarding FQ safety concerns, and pharmaceutical manufacturer responses regarding FQ safety concerns, with a specific focus on FQAD. Data include information presented by manufacturers, regulatory officials, and academic scientists at an FDA Joint Advisory Committee for Antimicrobials and Drug Risk and Safety meeting in 2015 (on FQ safety and efficacy), a meeting of the Pharmacovigilance Risk Advisory Committee (PRAC) of the European Medicines Agency in 2018 (on FQ safety), publicly disseminated notifications from the manufacturers, the FDA, and the European Medicines Agency (on the respective websites), and PubMed searches (MeSH terms: FQ name, ADRs, FQAD, neuropsychiatric toxicity, aortic dissection), the FDA's Adverse Event Reporting System (FAERS) database, and data reported by a National Cancer Institute R01 grant-supported pharmacovigilance program, the Southern Network on Adverse Reports (SONAR).

Protecting public health and patient safety from adverse drug reactions is incumbent upon drug manufacturers, the FDA, providers, and pharmacists. From Phase I studies through market approval, unexpected ADRs that occur infrequently and occasionally frequently become evident as more patients are exposed to drugs.

1.1.1 FQ Adverse Event Drug Label Warnings

FQs contain boxed warnings, the most serious type of drug label warnings. The boxed warnings indicate that FQs "have been associated with disabling and potentially irreversible serious adverse reactions that have occurred together," including tendinitis and tendon rupture, peripheral neuropathy, and central nervous system effects, which include psychiatric reactions. Additionally, boxed warnings warn that FQs may exacerbate muscle weakness in patients with myasthenia gravis. Finally, the boxed warnings explain that because FQs "have been associated with serious adverse reactions," they should be only used in patients who have no alternative treatment for uncomplicated urinary tract infection, acute bacterial exacerbation of chronic bronchitis, and acute bacterial sinusitis.

The "Warnings and Precautions" section of FQ labels also contains details of additional central nervous system adverse events, including psychiatric and neurological events, as well as a long list of other possible adverse events.

Despite these recommendations, a 2018 peer-reviewed article reported more than 6 million cases of FQs prescription outside the recommended administration protocol, with some cases not requiring antibiotic prescriptions at all [Kabbani].

1.1.2 FQ Drug Label Changes (See Table 1.1 for Levofloxacin Label Changes)

Since being approved by the FDA in 1998, FQ labels have gone through extensive changes, raising the question to the drug's safety from the time it was initially approved. Most of these changes occurred since 2006.

Table 1.1 Partial listing of Label Changes for levofloxacin (1998–2021)

Date of Levaquin label change	Levaquin label change
12/17/1998	Initial approved Levaquin label
9/08/2000	Changed label to include uncomplicated urinary tract infections as an approved use
12/18/2001	Added "Post-marketing surveillance reports indicate that this risk may be increased in patients receiving concomitant corticosteroids, especially in the elderly"
5/23/2003	Changed label to include chronic bacterial prostatitis as an approved use
3/05/2004	Added label language to indicate that Levaquin should only be used to treat or prevent infections that are proven or strongly suspected to be caused by bacteria
7/14/2004	Added "MDRSP (Multi-drug resistant Streptococcus pneumoniae) isolates are strains resistant to two or more of the following antibiotics: penicillin (MIC $\geq$ 2 µg/ml), 2nd generation cephalosporins, e.g., cefuroxime, macrolides, tetracyclines and trimethoprim/sulfamethoxazole"
9/14/2004	• Added "Peripheral Neuropathy: Rare cases of sensory or sensorimotor axonal polyneuropathy affecting small and/or large axons resulting in paresthesias, hypoesthesias, dysesthesias and weakness have been reported in patients receiving quinolones, including levofloxacin. Levofloxacin should be discontinued if the patient experiences symptoms of neuropathy including pain, burning, tingling, numbness, and/or weakness or other alterations of sensation including light touch, pain, temperature, position sense,

(continued)

Table 1.1 (continued)

Date of Levaquin label change	Levaquin label change
	and vibratory sensation in order to prevent the development of an irreversible condition"
	• Updated "Ruptures of the shoulder, hand, "or Achilles tendon, or other tendons" that required surgical repair or resulted in prolonged disability have been reported in patients receiving quinolones, including levofloxacin"
	• Updated "Torsades de pointes: Some quinolones, including levofloxacin, have been associated with prolongation of the QT interval on the electrocardiogram and infrequent cases of arrhythmia…"
	• Added "that peripheral neuropathies have been associated with levofloxacin use. If symptoms of peripheral neuropathy including pain, burning, tingling, numbness, and/or weakness develop, they should discontinue treatment and contact their physicians"
	• Added "Elderly patients may be more susceptible to drug-associated effects on the QT interval…"
	• Added "peripheral neuropathy, rhabdomyolysis," to the Post-marketing Adverse Events
11/04/2004	• Made changes to the following sections: DESCRIPTION, CLINICAL PHARMACOLOGY, and INDICATIONS AND USAGE
	• Revised the WARNINGS section to read, "in immature rats and dogs, the oral and intravenous administration of levofloxacin resulted in increased the incidence and severity of osteochondrosis. Histopathological examination of the weight-bearing joints of immature dogs dosed with levofloxacin revealed persistent lesions of the cartilage…"
	• Revised the PRECAUTIONS, DOSAGE AND ADMINISTRATION, HOW SUPPLIED, ANIMAL PHARMACOLOGY, and Patient Package Information sections
11/24/2004	• Added "Inhalational anthrax (post-exposure): To prevent the development of inhalational anthrax following exposure to Bacillus anthracis (See DOSAGE AND ADMINISTRATION and ADDITIONAL INFORMATION—INHALATIONAL ANTHRAX). Levofloxacin has not been tested in human for the post-exposure prevention of inhalation anthrax. However, plasma concentrations achieved in humans are reasonably likely to predict efficacy"
	• Made various other references to anthrax, as well"
8/04/2005	Updated dosing information
6/23/2006	• Made a number of changes to "CLINICAL PHARMACOLOGY/ MICROBIOLOGY" section
	• Re-worded information about anthrax in the INDICATIONS AND USAGE section
5/31/2007	Revised the "ADVERSE REACTIONS/Post-Marketing Adverse Reactions subsections of the "patient package insert for Levaquin to

(continued)

Table 1.1 (continued)

Date of Levaquin label change	Levaquin label change
	add new adverse reactions and reorganize the existing list of adverse reactions: Additional adverse events reported from worldwide post-marketing experience with levofloxacin include: allergic pneumonitis; hypersensitivity reactions sometimes fatal, including anaphylactic shock, anaphylactoid reaction, serum sickness, angioneurotic edema; dysphonia, abnormal EEG; encephalopathy; eosinophilia, erythema multiforme; StevensJohnson Syndrome; toxic epidermal necrolysis; peripheral neuropathy; rhabdomyolysis; muscle injury including rupture; tendon rupture; electrocardiogram QT prolonged; torsades de pointes; vasodilation; psychosis; paranoia; isolated reports of suicide attempts or suicidal ideation; multi-system organ failure; pseudomembraneous/C. difficile colitis; hepatitis; anosmia; ageusia; hypoacusis; dysphonia, vision disturbances including diplopia, visual acuity reduced, vision blurred, scotomata; leukocytoclastic vasculitis; photosensitivity reaction; acute renal failure; interstitial nephritis; eosinophilia; hemolytic anemia; leukopenia; pancytopenia; aplastic anemia; increased International Normalized Ratio (INR)/prothrombin time"
5/10/2007	• Added language in the WARNINGS section about "Clostridium difficile associated diarrhea (CDAD)" • Added in the PRECAUTIONS/ Information for Patients section "that diarrhea is a common problem caused by antibiotics which usually ends when the antibiotic is discontinued. Sometimes after starting treatment with antibiotics, patients can develop watery and bloody stools (with or without stomach cramps and fever) even as late as two or more months after having taken the last dose of the antibiotic…" • Added to the "Patient Package Insert/What are the possible side effects of LEVAQUIN? Diarrhea that usually ends after treatment is a common problem caused by antibiotics. A more serious form of diarrhea can occur during or up to 2 months after use of antibiotics…"
6/19/2007	• Updated the Hypersensitivity Reactions section to read, "Other serious and sometimes fatal events, some due to hypersensitivity, and some due to uncertain etiology, have been reported rarely in patients receiving therapy with quinolones, including Levaquin. These events may be severe and generally occur following the administration of multiple doses. Clinical manifestations may include one or more of the following: • fever, rash, or severe dermatologic reactions (e.g., toxic epidermal necrolysis, Stevens-Johnson Syndrome); • vasculitis; arthralgia; myalgia; serum sickness; • allergic pneumonitis; • interstitial nephritis; acute renal insufficiency or failure; • hepatitis; jaundice; acute hepatic necrosis or failure; • anemia, including hemolytic and aplastic; thrombocytopenia, including thrombotic thrombocytopenic purpura; leukopenia; agranulocytosis; pancytopenia; and/or other hematologic abnormalities. The drug should be discontinued

(continued)

Table 1.1 (continued)

Date of Levaquin label change	Levaquin label change
	immediately at the first appearance of a skin rash, jaundice, or any other sign of hypersensitivity and supportive measures instituted" • Revised the WARNINGS/Tendon Effects section to read, "Ruptures of the shoulder, hand, Achilles tendon, or other tendons that required surgical repair or resulted in prolonged disability have been reported in patients receiving quinolones, including levofloxacin. Post-marketing surveillance reports indicate that this risk may be is increased in patients receiving concomitant corticosteroids, especially the elderly" • Revised the PRECAUTIONS/Information for Patients section to read, "to discontinue LEVAQUIN treatment and inform their physician if they experience pain, inflammation, or rupture of a tendon, and to rest and refrain from exercise until the diagnosis of tendonitis or tendon rupture has been confidently excluded. The risk of serious tendon disorders is higher in those over 65 years of age, especially those on steroids • Added to the PRECAUTIONS/Information for Patients subsection following the last bulleted point: • "to inform their physician of any personal or family history of QTc prolongation or proarrhythmic conditions such as hypokalemia, bradycardia, or recent myocardial ischemia; if they are taking any class IA (quinidine, procainamide), or class III (amiodarone, sotalol) antiarrhythmic agents. Patients should notify their physicians if they have any symptoms of prolongation of the QTc interval, including prolonged heart palpitations or a loss of consciousness" • Revised the PRECAUTIONS/Geriatric Use section to read, "patients over 65 are at increased risk for developing severe tendon disorders including tendon rupture when being treated with a fluoroquinolone such as LEVAQUIN. This risk is further increased with age concomitant steroid therapy. Tendon rupture usually involves the Achilles, hand or shoulder tendons and can occur during therapy or up to a few months post completion of therapy. Caution should be used when prescribing levofloxacin to elderly patients especially those on corticosteroids. Patients should be informed of this potential side effect and advised to discontinue therapy and inform their physicians if any tendon symptoms occur" • Revised the ADVERSE REACTIONS/Post-Marketing Adverse Reactions section to include "hepatic failure (including fatal cases)" • Revised the Patient Package Insert section to read "What are possible side effects of Levaquin?: Pain, swelling, and tears of Achilles, Ruptures of shoulder, or hand, or Achilles tendons have been reported in patients receiving fluoroquinolones, including LEVAQUIN, for tendon effects is higher if you are over 65 years old, and especially if you are taking corticosteroids. If you develop pain, swelling, or rupture of a tendon you should stop taking LEVAQUIN, avoid exercise and strenuous use of the affected area, and contact your health care professional provider. In a few people, LEVAQUIN, like some other antibiotics, may produce a small

(continued)

Table 1.1 (continued)

Date of Levaquin label change	Levaquin label change
	effect on the heart that is seen on an electrocardiogram test. The rare heart problem is called QT prolongation and can cause an abnormal heartbeat and can be very dangerous. The chances of this event are increased in those with a family history of prolonged QT interval, low potassium (hypokalemia), and who are taking drugs to control heart rhythm, called class IA (quinidine, procainamide), or class III (amiodarone, sotalol) antiarrhythmic agents…."
9/14/2007	Added to the label, "treatment of complicated urinary tract infection and acute pyelonephritis with Levaquin 750 mg once daily for five days"
11/15/2007	Updated Use in Specific Populations section
11/16/2007	Updated "DOSAGE AND ADMINISTRATION section
12/13/2007	• Revised the WARNINGS AND PRECAUTIONS, Photosensitivity/Phototoxicity section to read, "moderate to severe phototoxicity reactions have been observed in patients exposed to direct sunlight while receiving drugs in this class… • Revised the ADVERSE REACTIONS, Serious and Otherwise Important Adverse Reactions section • Revised the ADVERSE REACTIONS, Post-Marketing Adverse Events section • Revised the PATIENT COUNSELING INFORMATION, FDA-Approved Patient Labeling/Patient Information, About Levaquin/What are possible side effects of Levaquin? section
4/16/2008	• Revised the HIGHLIGHTS/WARNINGS AND PRECAUTIONS section to read, "Hematologic (including agranulocytosis, thrombocytopenia), and renal toxicities may occur after multiple doses, Hepatotoxicity: Severe, and sometimes fatal, hepatotoxicity has been reported. Discontinue immediately if signs and symptoms of hepatitis occur" • Revised the HIGHLIGHTS/USE IN SPECIFIC POPULATIONS/Geriatrics section to read, "Geriatrics: Severe hepatotoxicity has been reported. The majority of reports describe patients 65 years of age or older. May have increased risk of tendon disorders (including rupture), especially with concomitant corticosteroid use. May be more susceptible to prolongation of the QT interval" • Revised the WARNINGS AND PRECAUTIONS section to read, "Hepatotoxicity Post-marketing reports of severe hepatotoxicity (including acute hepatitis and fatal events) have been received for patients treated with LEVAQUIN®. No evidence of serious drug-associated hepatotoxicity was detected in clinical trials of over 7,000 patients. Severe hepatotoxicity generally occurred within 14 days of initiation of therapy and most cases occurred within 6 days. Most cases of severe hepatotoxicity were not associated with hypersensitivity…" • Revised the Patient Counseling Information • Revised the ADVERSE REACTIONS section to read, "Serious and Otherwise Important Adverse Reactions" address Hypersensitivity

(continued)

Table 1.1 (continued)

Date of Levaquin label change	Levaquin label change
	Reactions, Other Serious and Sometimes Fatal Reactions, Hepatotoxicity, Tendon Effects, Central Nervous System Effects, Clostridium difficile-Associated Diarrhea, Peripheral Neuropathy, Prolongation of the QT Interval, Musculoskeletal Disorders in Pediatric Patients, Blood Glucose Disturbances, Photosensitivity/Phototoxicity, Development of Drug Resistant Bacteria • Revised the USE IN SPECIFIC POPULATIONS/Geriatric Use section • Revised the PATIENT COUNSELING INFORMATION, Serious and Potentially Serious Adverse Reactions section • Revised the PATIENT COUNSELING INFORMATION, FDA-Approved Patient Labeling/Patient Information About Levaquin/What are possible side effects of Levaquin? Section • Made "editorial changes throughout the label"
10/03/2008	• Added a Boxed Warning to the Highlights and to the beginning of the Full Prescribing Information section as follows: "WARNING: Fluoroquinolones, including LEVAQUIN®, are associated with an increased risk of tendonitis and tendon rupture in all ages. This risk is further increased in older patients usually over 60 years of age, in patients taking corticosteroid drugs, and in patients with kidney, heart or lung transplants • Revised other label sections related to risk of tendonitis and tendon rupture
2/25/2011	• Added to the Boxed Warning, "Fluoroquinolones, including LEVAQUIN®, may exacerbate muscle weakness in persons with myasthenia gravis. Avoid LEVAQUIN® in patients with known history of myasthenia gravis • Added to the WARNINGS AND PRECAUTIONS section, "Exacerbation of myasthenia gravis Fluoroquinolones, including LEVAQUIN®, have neuromuscular blocking activity and may exacerbate muscle weakness in persons with myasthenia gravis. Postmarketing serious adverse events, including deaths and requirement for ventilatory support, have been associated with fluoroquinolone use in persons with myasthenia gravis. Avoid LEVAQUIN® in patients with known history of myasthenia gravis • Updated the Patient Counseling Information related to myasthenia gravis warnings • Made other miscellaneous label updates
4/27/2012	• Added "1.14 Plague LEVAQUIN® is indicated for treatment of plague, including pneumonic and septicemic plague, due to Yersinia pestis (Y. pestis) and prophylaxis for plague in adults and pediatric patients, 6 months of age and older. Efficacy studies of LEVAQUIN® could not be conducted in humans with plague for ethical and feasibility reasons. Therefore, approval of this indication was based on an efficacy study conducted in animals" • Made other miscellaneous label updates
8/14/2013	Revised the ADVERSE REACTIONS, Postmarketing Experience section

(continued)

Table 1.1 (continued)

Date of Levaquin label change	Levaquin label change
7/26/2016	• Revised Box Warning to read, "Fluoroquinolones, including LEVAQUIN®, have been associated with disabling and potentially irreversible serious adverse reactions that have occurred together (5.1), including: o Tendinitis and tendon rupture (5.2) o Peripheral neuropathy (5.3) o Central nervous system effects (5.4) Discontinue LEVAQUIN immediately and avoid the use of fluoroquinolones, including LEVAQUIN, in patients who experience any of these serious adverse reactions (5.1) • Fluoroquinolones, including LEVAQUIN®, may exacerbate muscle weakness in patients with myasthenia gravis. Avoid LEVAQUIN® in patients with a known history of myasthenia gravis [see Warnings and Precautions (5.5)]. • Because fluoroquinolones, including LEVAQUIN, have been associated with serious adverse reactions (5.1–5.14), reserve LEVAQUIN for use in patients who have no alternative treatment options for the following indications: o Uncomplicated urinary tract infection (1.12) o Acute bacterial exacerbation of chronic bronchitis (1.13) o Acute bacterial sinusitis (1.14)" • Revised the WARNINGS AND PRECAUTIONS section to read, "5.1 Disabling and Potentially Irreversible Serious Adverse Reactions Including Tendinitis and Tendon Rupture, Peripheral Neuropathy, and Central Nervous System Effects Fluoroquinolones, including LEVAQUIN, have been associated with disabling and potentially irreversible serious adverse reactions from different body systems that can occur together in the same patient. Commonly seen adverse reactions include tendinitis, tendon rupture, arthralgia, myalgia, peripheral neuropathy, and central nervous system effects (hallucinations, anxiety, depression, insomnia, severe headaches, and confusion). These reactions can occur within hours to weeks after starting LEVAQUIN. Patients of any age or without pre-existing risk factors have experienced these adverse reactions [see Warnings and Precautions (5.2, 5.3, 5.4)] • Revised Patient Counseling Information to read, "Disabling and Potentially Irreversible Serious Adverse Reactions That May Occur Together: Inform patients that disabling and potentially irreversible serious adverse reactions, including tendinitis and tendon rupture, peripheral neuropathies, and central nervous system effects, have been associated with use of LEVAQUIN and may occur together in the same patient. Inform patients to stop taking LEVAQUIN immediately if they experience an adverse reaction and to call their healthcare provider. Discontinue LEVAQUIN immediately at the first signs or symptoms of any serious adverse reaction. In addition, avoid the use of fluoroquinolones, including LEVAQUIN, in patients who have experienced any of these serious adverse reactions associated with fluoroquinolones"
2/08/2017	• No changes were made to the Medication Guide •Revised WARNINGS AND PRECAUTIONS, Central Nervous System section to "state the risk of completed suicide, especially in

(continued)

Table 1.1 (continued)

Date of Levaquin label change	Levaquin label change
	patients with a medical history of depression or an underlying risk factor for depression" • Revised ADVERSE REACTIONS, Postmarketing Experience section to "include completed suicide, Acute Generalized Exanthematous Pustulosis (AGEP), and fixed drug eruptions" • Revised MEDICATION GUIDE was to clarify language regarding skin rash"
10/18/2018	• Revised the Central Nervous Effects section, as follows: "Psychiatric Adverse Reactions Fluoroquinolones, including LEVAQUIN®, have been associated with an increased risk of psychiatric adverse reactions, including: toxic psychoses, hallucinations, or paranoia; depression, or suicidal thoughts; anxiety, agitation, restlessness, or nervousness; confusion, delirium, disorientation, or disturbances in attention; insomnia or nightmares; memory impairment. Attempted or completed suicide have been reported, especially in patients with a medical history of depression, or an underlying risk factor for depression. These reactions may occur following the first dose. If these reactions occur in patients receiving LEVAQUIN®, discontinue LEVAQUIN® and institute appropriate measures. Central Nervous System Adverse Reactions Fluoroquinolones, including LEVAQUIN®, have been associated with an increased risk of seizures (convulsions), increased intracranial pressure (including pseudotumor cerebri), tremors, and lightheadedness. As with other fluoroquinolones, LEVAQUIN® should be used with caution in patients with a known or suspected central nervous system (CNS) disorder that may predispose them to seizures or lower the seizure threshold (e.g., severe cerebral arteriosclerosis, epilepsy) or in the presence of other risk factors that may predispose them to seizures or lower the seizure threshold (e.g., certain drug therapy, renal dysfunction). If these reactions occur in patients receiving LEVAQUIN®, discontinue LEVAQUIN® and institute appropriate measures [see Adverse Reactions (6), Drug Interactions" • Added, "Blood Glucose Disturbances Fluoroquinolones, including LEVAQUIN®, have been associated with disturbances of blood glucose, including symptomatic hyperglycemia and hypoglycemia, usually in diabetic patients receiving concomitant treatment with an oral hypoglycemic agent (e.g., glyburide) or with insulin. In these patients, careful monitoring of blood glucose is recommended. Severe cases of hypoglycemia resulting in coma or death have been reported. If a hypoglycemic reaction occurs in a patient being treated with LEVAQUIN®, discontinue LEVAQUIN® and initiate appropriate therapy immediately (see Adverse Reactions (6.2), Drug Interactions (7.3) and Patient Counseling Information [17]) • No changes were made to the Patient Counseling Information or Medication Guide sections"
6/28/2019	• Revised the "HIGHLIGHTS OF PRESCRIBING INFORMATION, USE IN SPECIFIC POPULATIONS Pregnancy, Lactation section • Revised the PATIENT COUNSELING INFORMATION section

(continued)

Table 1.1 (continued)

Date of Levaquin label change	Levaquin label change
	• Revised the CLINICAL PHARMACOLOGY, Clinical Microbiology section • Revised the DOSAGE AND ADMINISTRATION, Important Administration Instructions section • Updated the Medication Guide • Made "minor editorial changes and clarifications throughout
6/22/2020	• Revised the HIGHLIGHTS OF PRESCRIBING INFORMATION and the USE IN SPECIFIC POPULATIONS, Lactation sections to "provide for the risk benefit assessment of Levaquin tablets for inhalational anthrax (post-exposure)" • Updated the Medication Guide • Made "minor editorial changes" throughout

1.1.3 FDA Reports of FQ Adverse Events

The following highlights FQ adverse events reported to the FDA Adverse Events Reporting System (FAERS) data, by category.

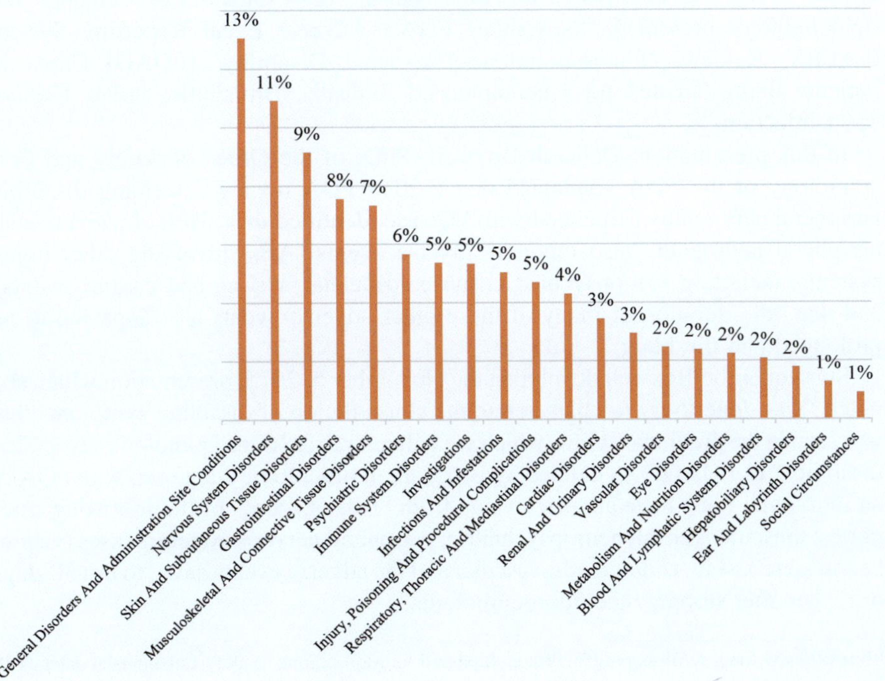

FQ-associated deaths have also been reported to the FDA. The following high-lights FQ death adverse events reported to the FAERS, reported from 2000 to 2020.

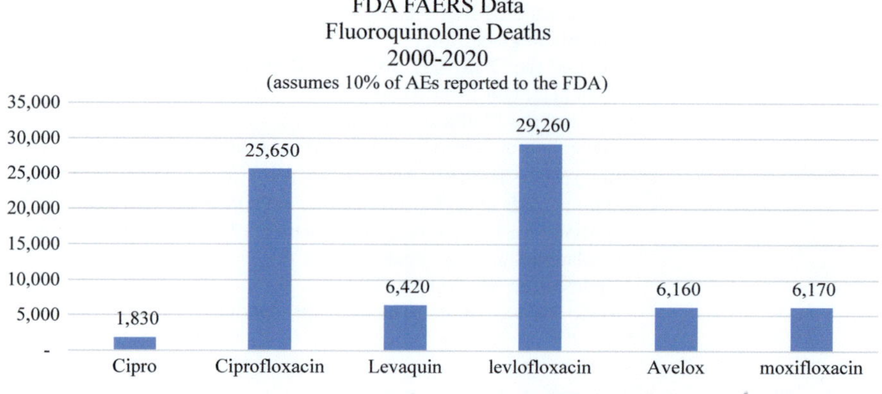

1.1.4 November 5, 2015, FDA Advisory Committee Meeting Identifies FQAD

On November 5, 2015, the FDA held a Joint Meeting of the Antimicrobial Drugs Advisory Committee and the Drug Safety and Risk Management Advisory Committee. At this meeting, Debra Boxwell from the FDA Office of Surveillance and Epidemiology presented, "November FDA's Adverse Event Reporting System (FAERS) Review: 'Fluoroquinolone-Associated Disability' (FQAD) Cases in Patients Being Treated for Uncomplicated Sinusitis, Bronchitis, and/or Urinary Tract Infection."[1]

In this presentation, Deborah Boxwell, PhD, of the Office of Safety and Epidemiology of the FDA, explained that a 2013 FDA review describing disabling peripheral neuropathy associated with FQs use identified that "76% of patients with peripheral neuropathy also reported adverse events (AEs) involving other organ systems, including neuropsychiatric, musculoskeletal, vision, and cardiac events" and that "the duration of many of these other adverse events also appeared to be prolonged and disabling."

Subsequently, Boxwell developed the November 5, 2015, presentation which she noted "was done to try to characterize the constellation of disabling symptoms that was seen in the previous review, which we will refer to as 'fluoroquinolone-associated disability,' or FQAD." As defined by Boxwell, in order to be diagnosed with FQAD, an individual must have adverse events from "two or more" of the following categories: musculoskeletal, neuropsychiatric, peripheral nervous system, senses (vision, hearing, etc.), skin, and/or cardiovascular and the adverse events have "to last 30 days or longer after stopping the fluoroquinolone."

---

[1] https://www.fda.gov/files/about%20fda/published/Fluoroquinolone- Safety-Labeling-Updates-%28 PDF—1.15MB%29.pdf.

1.1.5   November 5, 2015, FDA Advisory Committee Votes

After the presentation at the FDA Advisory Committee meeting by Boxwell, patients injured by FQs, and FQ drug company representatives, the FDA Advisory Committee voted overwhelmingly that existing FQ drug labels were not adequate.

1. Do the benefits and risks of the systemic fluoroquinolone antibacterial drugs support the current labeled indication for the treatment of acute bacterial sinusitis (ABS)?	NO: 21 YES: 0 ABSTAIN: 0
2. Do the benefits and risks of the systemic fluoroquinolone antibacterial drugs support the current labeled indication for the treatment of acute bacterial exacerbation of chronic bronchitis in patients who have chronic obstructive pulmonary disease (ABECB-COPD)?	NO: 18 YES: 2 ABSTAIN: 1
3. VOTE: Do the benefits and risks of the systemic fluoroquinolone antibacterial drugs support the current labeled indication for the treatment of uncomplicated urinary tract infection (uUTI)?	NO: 20 YES: 1 ABSTAIN: 0

1.1.6   Boxwell FDA FQ Data Compared with Social Media FQ Reports

Boxwell's November 5, 2015, FQAD presentation reviewed only a small subset of FQs adverse event reports submitted to the FDA. Specifically, Boxwell only analyzed cases identified as having a disability and only having been treated for urinary tract infection, sinusitis, and bronchitis.

SONAR, in conjunction with an extensive community of individuals injured by FQs, has reviewed FQ research, FQ FDA adverse events data, and FQ patient narratives for the past decade. Based on these reviews, SONAR considered that FQAD may be more extensive than implied by the Boxwell Study. This research review compares the results of Boxwell's data, as included in her November 5, 2015, FQAD presentation, with analysis an of patient narratives shared on social media sites, the "FQ Community Study," related to individuals who reportedly experienced FQ adverse events.

The Boxwell Study examined 1,122 cases of individuals who reported disability after being treated with an oral FQ for a urinary tract infection, sinusitis, or bronchitis, based on FDA reports of FQ adverse events submitted to the FDA from November 1, 1997. to May 30, 2015.

On the other hand, the social media FQ Community Study evaluated 223 cases of individuals who reported FQ adverse events after being treated for a wide range of diagnoses and included both oral and IV FQs. The FQ Community Study analyzed all patient narratives that contained enough information to create a record. Importantly, the FQ Community Study stories were collected through Facebook groups prior to 2015 and, therefore, were written prior to Boxwell defining FQAD.

Of 1,122 disability reports evaluated by Boxwell, it was determined that 178 cases met the definition of FQAD, as Boxwell defined at the November 5, 2015, FDA Advisory Committee meeting; 944 did not meet the FQAD definition.

Of 223 narratives submitted to online social media websites describing the experiences of those with fluoroquinolone adverse event, 218 met the definition of FQAD, 4 did not meet the FQAD definition, and 1 case could not be determined.

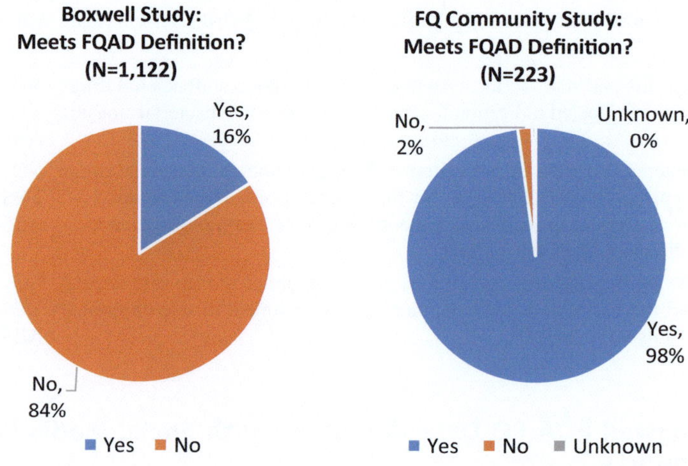

Histories submitted by individuals to online social media sites were generally more detailed. Notably, FDA reports were often initial reports submitted immediately after patients recognized adverse events following FQs utilization, and therefore, did not include reporting of potentially extensive ADR symptoms which develop or are recognized over time.

Importantly, the FQ Community Study indicates that even in the absence of the FDA's description of FQAD which was not defined until 2015, 98% of those who reported FQ adverse events on social media met the definition of FQAD when analyzed retrospectively.

A recent conversation with members of the online FQ communities has brought to light the necessity to expand Bowell's diagnostic criteria for FQAD. Indeed, the results of a study by Dr. Bove at Bucknell University (Lewisburg, PA) revealed that approximately 67% of the 306 participants interviewed have a high likelihood of suffering from functional gastrointestinal disorders (FGD), with higher percentages reported from patients that utilized ciprofloxacin or levofloxacin (72% and 76%, respectively).[2] Interestingly, there seems to be no correlation between the likelihood of FGD incidence and FQs dosage or length of administration. Since patients with pre-existing gastrointestinal issues and/or diagnoses were excluded from the study, and considering that the study assessed the presence of gastrointestinal symptoms in the last 12 months, these results strongly highlight the necessity to include FGD in the diagnostic criteria for FQAD. The researchers leading the study hypothesize that the possible cause behind these motility issues is the antagonistic activity of FQs against gamma-aminobutyric acid $(GABA)_A$ receptors in concert with the agonistic

---

[2] https://www.mdpi.com/1648-9144/57/12/1371.

activity to N-methyl-D-aspartate (NMDA) receptors, both of which are key regulators of the motor branch of the vagus nerve, the parasympathetic cranial nerve regulating gastrointestinal function [Freeman]. In support of this idea, the same research group has recently shown at the Susquehanna Valley Undergraduate Research Symposium of 2021 that rats treated with ciprofloxacin show a significant acceleration of gastrointestinal motility compared to naïve rats. Hence, the possibility that FQs may permanently affect vagal activity cannot be excluded.

1.1.7 Gender

Of 178 FQAD cases in the Boxwell Study, 40 were male and 138 were female. The FQ Community Study included 45 males and 178 females who met the FQAD definition.

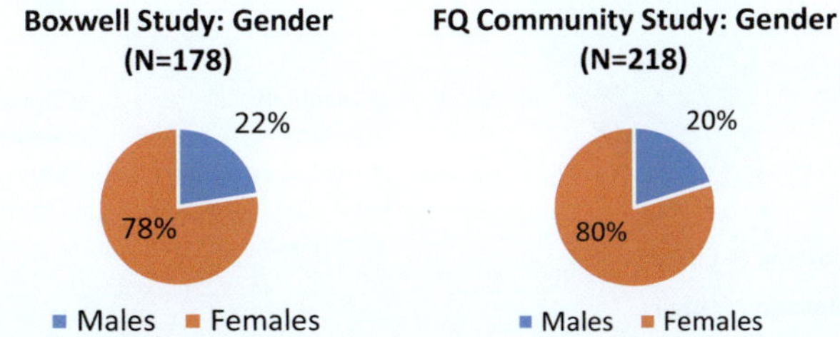

Although more females were included in both studies, the FDA study found similar gender differences even when excluding urinary tract infections (which are overwhelmingly female-associated).

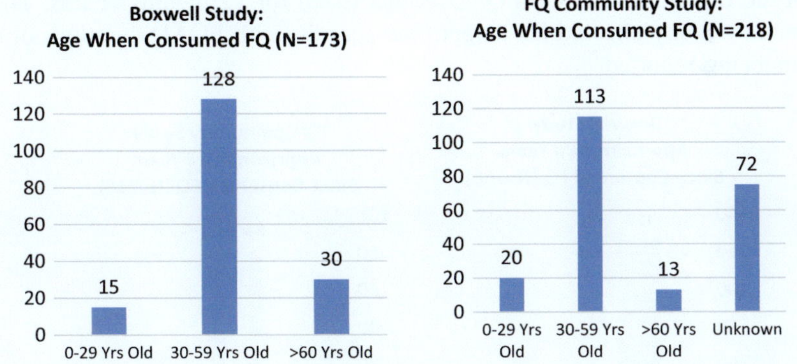

In the Boxwell Study, two individuals are reported to have been under the age of 18.

1.1.8 Specific FQs

FQAD individuals in both the Boxwell Study and the FQ Community Study had received primarily Levaquin/levofloxacin, Cipro/ciprofloxacin, and/or Avelox/moxifloxacin.

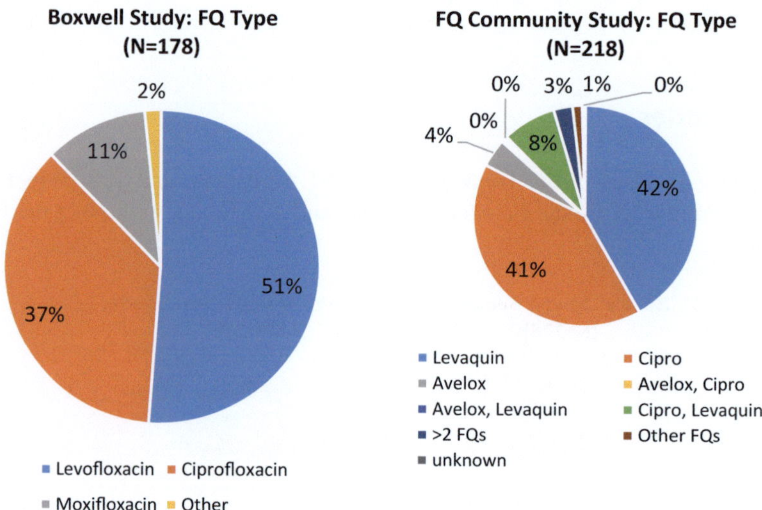

1.1.9 Duration of FQAD

All of the Boxwell-identified FQAD events lasted for 12 months or less. The FQ Community Study allowed for longer time periods, with FQAD durations of up to 9 years being reported.

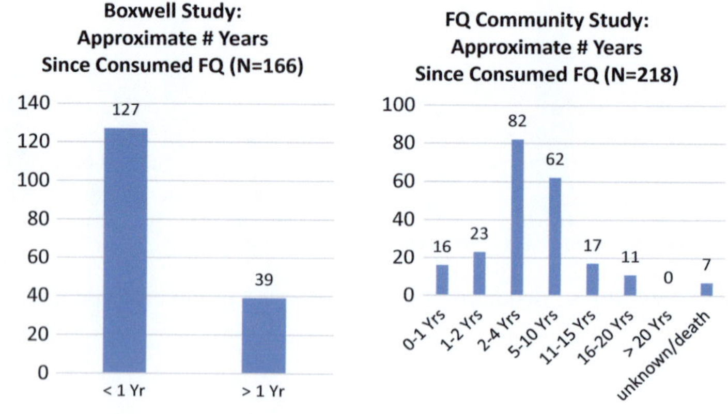

1.1.10   FQAD: Reasons for Which FQ was Prescribed

The Boxwell study reviewed a small subset of FQ adverse event reports submitted to the FDA which were identified as having a disability of 12 months or less, plus having been treated for urinary tract infection, sinusitis, and/or bronchitis.

The FQ Community Study reviewed cases of individuals who were prescribed FQs for a wide range of diagnoses.

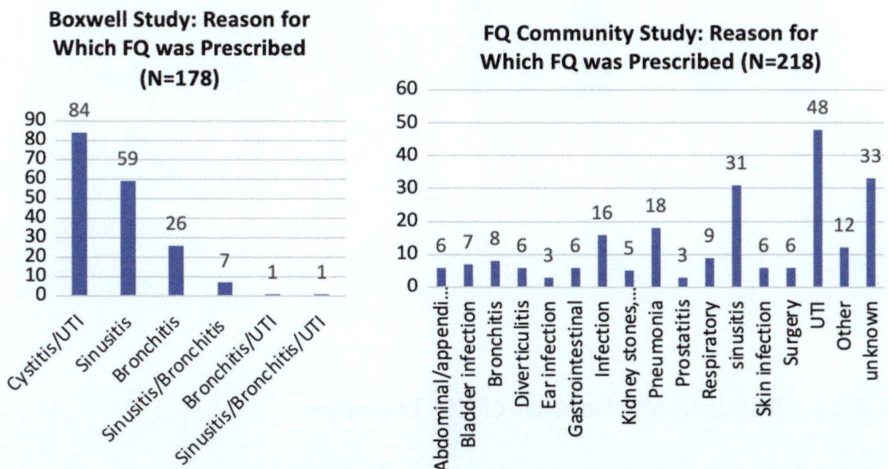

The FQ Community Study indicates that FQAD may result from taking FQs for a wide range of clinical diagnoses and is not limited to affecting only individuals who received FQs for treatment of urinary tract infections, sinusitis, or bronchitis.

1.1.11   FQAD Specific Events

Although the FQ Community Study did not evaluate the specific categories of FQAD adverse events, the Boxwell Study did.

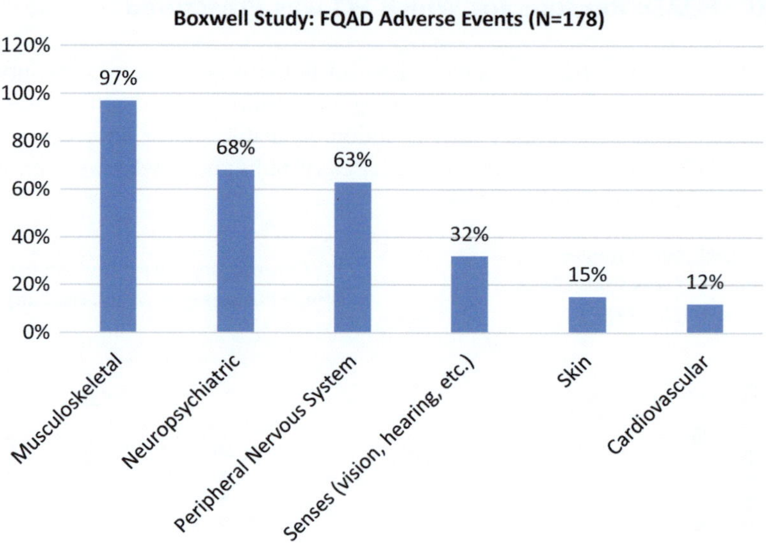

1.1.12 Possible Mechanism of FQ Toxicities

On April 17, 2013, the FDA disseminated a Pharmacovigilance Review that discusses a possible mechanism of action related to FQ adverse events: mitochondrial toxicity. This review describes that "in vitro studies in drug-treated mammalian cells found that nalidixic acid and ciprofloxacin caused a loss of mitochondrial DNA (mtDNA), resulting in a decrease of mitochondrial respiration and an arrest in cell growth." The review further explains that "mitochondrial conditions that are due to an insufficiency of ATP, especially in organs that rely on mitochondria for their energy source, include developmental disorders of the brain, optic neuropathy, neuropathic pain, hearing loss, muscle weakness, cardiomyopathy, and lactic acidosis [6]. Neurodegenerative diseases, like Parkinson's, Alzheimer's, and amyotrophic lateral sclerosis (ALS) have been associated with the loss of neurons due to oxidative stress."

FAERS data identifies adverse events related to neurodegenerative diseases (which is consistent with mitochondrial toxicity). In the FDA FAERS data from 2000 to 2020, there have been 73 cases which reported an FQ adverse event with the term "Parkinson's, 13 cases which reported an FQ adverse event with the term "ALS," 7 cases which reported an FQ adverse event with the term "Alzheimer's," 153 cases which reported an FQ adverse event with the term "multiple sclerosis," and 11 cases which reported "neurodegenerative disorder". There are, however, thousands of cases which have reported FQ adverse events describing symptoms similar to those suffered by individuals with Parkinson's, ALS, and Alzheimer's, some of which are included in the FQ top 20 FAERS adverse events documented in charts elsewhere in this document. Because the FDA acknowledges that only 10%

of adverse events are reported to the FDA, the following indicates the estimated actual neurodegenerative adverse events, based on the FDA FAERS data.

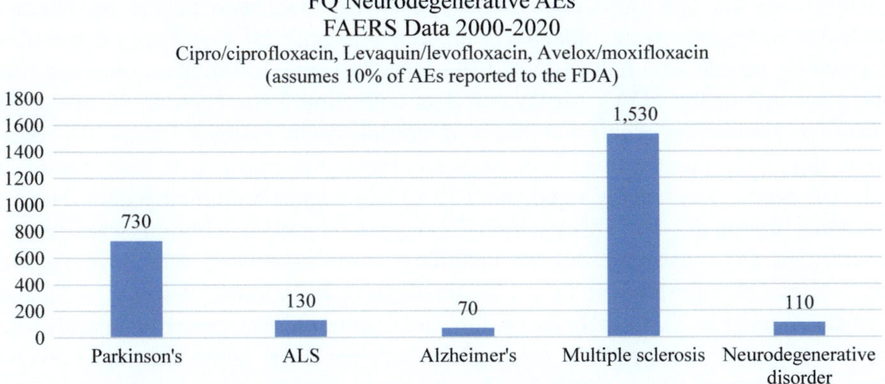

1.1.13   Another Possible Pathophysiologic Mechanism: Matrix Metalloproteinase Toxicity

FQs upregulate matrix metalloproteinases (MMPs), enzymes which degrade collagen, especially collagen I and III. This is a mechanism by which FQs are hypothesized to rupture tendons. FQs upregulate MMPs, including MMP-1, MMP-2, and MMP-13, resulting in reductions in the diameter and amount of type I collagen fibrils. FQs also cause degenerative changes in tendon cells with vacuole formation, organelle dilatation, and apoptosis. [Tsai] FQs can cause degenerative changes in tendon cells that lead to resultant vacuole formation.

Collagen and elastin are primary extracellular matrix components of the aortic wall. In a human in vitro study, human aortic myofibroblasts were isolated from nine patients with aortopathy undergoing elective ascending aortic resection. [Guzzardi]. The study assessed the capacity for extracellular matrix degradation in FQ exposed cells by multiplex analysis of secreted MMPs relative to tissue inhibitors of matrix metalloproteinases (TIMPs). Direct evaluation of extracellular matrix degradation was investigated. Aortic cellular collagen-1 expression increased following FQ exposure as noted by immunoblotting and immunofluorescent staining and cell apoptosis, and necrosis.

Furthermore, Reviglio et al. found MMP-1, MMP-2, MMP-8, and MMP-9 expression at 48 h in undebrided corneal epithelium groups treated with the topical FQs [Reviglio].

1.1.14 FQ-Associated Peripheral Neuropathy

In 2001, a survey of persons with FQ-associated peripheral neuropathy was reported by the late Jay Cohen MD. The survey had been posted on internet websites and cases were obtained with the assistance of members of websites formed by people who had sustained FQ-related events. Information obtained met the standards of the FDA's MedWatch data collection form. Overall, 36 of the 45 cases reported severe events that involved multiple organ systems. Symptoms lasted more than three months in 71% of cases and more than one year in 58%. Onset of adverse events was usually rapid, with 15 (33%) events beginning within 24 h of initiating treatment, 26 (58%) within 72 h, and 38 (84%) within 1 week. Sixty courses of FQs were prescribed, including cases associated with levofloxacin ($n = 33$ cases), ciprofloxacin ($n = 11$), ofloxacin ($n = 6$), lomefloxacin ($n = 1$), and trovafloxacin ($n = 1$). In eight cases, the same antibiotic was prescribed twice. The survey suggested a possible association between FQs antibiotics and severe, long-term adverse effects involving the peripheral nervous system and other organ systems. The severity of these cases may have reflected a different population than typically reported adverse events to pharmaceutical companies or to the FDA, which often originate from healthcare providers. The survey was one of the first papers to document the wide range of symptoms observed in persons with levofloxacin-associated neurologic toxicity. [Cohen].

1.1.15 Levaquin Clinical Trials Completed Prior to FDA Approval in 1997

A number of Levaquin clinical trials, as posted on the FDA website, were considered by the clinical trial reviewers to have "significant flaws". Some aspects were described as "confusing" or "troubling". Some of the trials were considered to have "significant flaws in the protocol design" and "significant flaws in protocol implementation," while some were considered to have clinical assessment categories which were "inappropriate". A clinical trial reviewer considered one Levaquin clinical trial to be "quite confusing from the clinical microbiology perspective" and said it contained "troubling" variations. In addition, it was noted that "some of the proposed quality control parameters simply do not make sense."

1.1.16 2001 FDA FQ Review

In 2001, the FDA's Office of Surveillance and Epidemiology published its first review on fluoroquinolone toxicity. This review was conducted in response to a patient contacting the FDA. The review, "Office of Safety and Epidemiology (OSE) Post-marketing Safety Review: Peripheral Neuropathy with Levofloxacin.

30 Apr 2001," identified 28 cases of peripheral neuropathy associated with levofloxacin. It found that peripheral neuropathy lasted as long as 2 years after patients received levofloxacin.

1.1.17   2003 FDA FQ Review

In 2003, the FDA wrote a second review on FQ-associated neuropathy, again conducted by the Office of Surveillance and Epidemiology, "Post-marketing Safety Review: Prolonged Peripheral Neuropathies with Fluoroquinolones." (Sally et al. 06 June 2003) This review described 108 cases of peripheral neuropathy associated with ciprofloxacin, levofloxacin, and/or ofloxacin. Thirty-four of the 108 cases reported peripheral neuropathy at time periods of a year or more after the drug had been discontinued, suggesting the potential irreversibility of the condition. The review recommended that peripheral neuropathy be added to the ciprofloxacin and levofloxacin labels.

1.1.18   2008 FDA Pediatric Levofloxacin Review

September 29, 2008, the FDA Division of Pharmacovigilance II DPVII completed a review of levofloxacin post-marketing adverse drug events in the pediatric population. The DPVII "concluded that the overall safety profile of levofloxacin in pediatrics appeared similar to adults without new serious unlabeled adverse events," noting that "musculoskeletal events, primarily arthralgia, were the most frequently reported events and represented the predominant adverse events reported among pediatric users. Central nervous system events were also reported in pediatric cases and were most often seizure, abnormal behavior, confusion, hallucination, and panic attack."

1.1.19   2010 Pfizer Report

In 2010, toxicologist Yvonne Will and her colleagues at Pfizer reported on an assay to detect mitochondrial damage early in drug development. (Nadanaciva et al., 2010) They found that some antibiotics affected mitochondria and others did not. Every FQs they tested damaged mitochondria in human liver cells, having what the researchers described as "a strong effect" at therapeutic concentrations. Will cautioned, however, that it was not possible to extrapolate from that result to clinical outcomes.

1.1.20   2011 Levaquin Postmarketing Review

On July 13, 2011, DPV II completed an updated review of levofloxacin post-marketing adverse events in accordance with the Pediatric Research Equity Act (PREA) 0.3 the focus of this review was reports of pediatric death and serious unlabeled adverse events with levofloxacin. The review concluded that the adverse events reported in children were similar to those reported in adults, primarily describing musculoskeletal and central nervous system events, both of which were adequately reflected in labeling. No new or significant adverse events in pediatric patients exposed to levofloxacin were identified.

1.1.21   2013 FDA Review

In 2013, a PubMed search on FQ-associated neuropathy was conducted by FDA employees. The search, undertaken by FDA's Office of Safety and Epidemiology (OSA) on November 12, 2012, identified 37 published articles related to FQ-associated neurotoxicity. After a review of titles and abstracts, 16 were deemed relevant and were further reviewed. Of these, eight provided adequate case descriptions. Citations in these eight articles identified two additional relevant articles, and an additional publication was identified through an incidental finding from another search. Overall, 91 cases of FQ-associated neuropathy were described in the literature. After excluding 45 cases considered of dubious quality by the OSA reviewer, 46 cases with higher quality data remained. Of these, 20 case reports described a temporal relationship and a positive de-challenge. Many cases were confounded, but the association with an FQ remained plausible. In at least one case, the neuropathy (carpal tunnel syndrome) was a result of tendonitis, a known complication of FQs. Most cases described in the literature reported resolution of symptoms. Of the 46 cases forming the core of this analysis, there was only one report (Hedenmalm and Spigset) where symptoms lasted "somewhat more than 1 year". Based on this literature review, the FDA concluded that there appeared to be good evidence for an association between the use of FQ and the development of peripheral neuropathy. Though one person developed symptoms of neuropathy after 5 months of treatment for osteomyelitis, most other patients developed symptoms of neuropathy within a few days after initiation of the drug. Over 20 cases described the resolution of symptoms after discontinuation of the drug. There was one credible report of symptoms extending beyond a year.

In the 2013 FDA review, the FDA noted that peer-reviewed publications supported the mitochondrial dysfunction theory of FQ-associated toxicity. The mechanisms underlying the effects of antibiotics in mammalian systems, however, are unclear. Some scientists suggest that bactericidal antibiotics induce the formation of toxic reactive oxygen species (ROS) in bacteria. Kalghatgi et al. showed that clinically relevant doses of bactericidal antibiotics-quinolones, aminoglycosides, and β-lactams-caused mitochondrial dysfunction and Reactive Oxygen Species (ROS) overproduction in mammalian cells. [Lawrence] It was demonstrated that these bactericidal antibiotic-induced effects led to oxidative damage to DNA, proteins, and membrane lipids. In the Lawrence study, mice treated with bactericidal antibiotics exhibited elevated oxidative stress markers in the blood, oxidative tissue damage, and up-regulated expression of key genes involved in antioxidant defense mechanisms, which points to the potential physiological relevance of these antibiotic effects. Deleterious effects of bactericidal antibiotics were alleviated in cell culture and in mice by the administration of the antioxidant N-acetyl-l-cysteine or prevented by preferential use of bacteriostatic antibiotics. This study highlighted the role of antibiotics in the production of oxidative tissue damage in mammalian cells.

In the 2013 review, the FDA highlighted mitochondrial toxicity as a possible mechanism for fluoroquinolone-associated toxicity. It was noted that FQs act by inhibiting DNA gyrase and bacterial topoisomerase IV, both of which are members of the topoisomerase type IIA subfamily. FQs affect mammalian topoisomerase II, particularly in mitochondria. In vitro studies in drug-related mammalian cells found that nalidixic acid and ciprofloxacin cause a loss of mitochondrial DNA causing a decrease in mitochondrial respiration and cell growth arrest. Mitochondrial conditions that are due to insufficient ATP, especially in organs that rely on mitochondria for energy, include developmental disorders of the brain, optic neuropathy, neuropathic pain, hearing loss, muscle weakness, cardiomyopathy, and lactic acidosis. Neurodegenerative diseases like Parkinson's, Alzheimer's, and amyotrophic lateral sclerosis have been associated with neuron loss due to oxidative stress [Rawj]. Ciprofloxacin has been reported to affect mammalian topoisomerase II, particularly in mitochondria. In vitro studies in drug-treated mammalian cells found that nalidixic acid and ciprofloxacin caused a loss of mitochondrial DNA, resulting in a decrease in mitochondrial regeneration and cell growth arrest. Additional analyses found protein-linked double-stranded DNA breaks in the mitochondrial DNA, resulting in a decrease in the mitochondrial DNA from ciprofloxacin-treated cells. This suggests that ciprofloxacin can target topoisomerase II activity in the mitochondria. An oxidative phosphorylation system found on the inner membrane of mitochondria provides 95% of the ATP requirements of the cell. Mitochondrial respiratory chains are major producers of oxidative stress [Fang]. This occurs when there is greater production of reactive oxygen species than anti-oxidative processes. About 1–4% of the oxygen reacting with the respiratory chain is incompletely reduced to superoxide radical ions, hydrogen peroxide, lipid peroxides, and other free radicals. Under normal circumstances, there is prevention or removal of ROS so that cellular damage is avoided. This includes lipid peroxidation, mitochondrial DNA mutations, and DNA strand breaks. If this does not occur, even more oxidative damage occurs. One human prospective study was done to evaluate oxidative stress among patients taking different doses of ciprofloxacin, levofloxacin, and gatifloxacin for five days for urinary tract infections [Talia]. Superoxide dismutase, glutathione, plasma anti-oxidant status, and lipid peroxides were evaluated in 52 patients. Ciprofloxacin causes a significant increase in lipid peroxide levels from the first to the fifth day. There were significant decreases in superoxide dismutase and glutathione. Similar results were noted for levofloxacin. The study showed how increased lipid peroxides can quickly overwhelm plasma antioxidants, leading to impaired cell integrity and cell death.

1.1.22 2014—Present Media Reports Regarding FQs

Since 2014, Drs. Bennett and Martin of the SONAR project at the University of South Carolina have communicated with reporters from across the country on more than 50 local news stories exposing the dangers of FQ antibiotics. These stories featured interviews with local residents who suffer from FQ toxicity. An FQ story from Atlanta by Jim Strickland received a Regional Emmy Award in 2014 and a second FQ story from Cleveland's Ron Regan also received a Regional Emmy Award.

1.1.23 2014 FDA Advisory Committee Comments

In August 2014, Dr. Martin submitted comments for September 23, 2014, FDA Advisory Committee focused on levofloxacin use in children. Based on FDA briefing materials for this meeting, approximately 100,000 children had already been prescribed levofloxacin even though the FDA has only approved the drug to treat anthrax and the plague in children. Dr. Martin requested that the FDA consider restricting levofloxacin use in the pediatric setting based on the FDA's FAERS data.

FDA's presentation, "Full Safety and Drug Utilization Review Provided in Background Materials Levaquin (levofloxacin) Pediatric Advisory Committee September 23, 2014" states that "the only labeled indications for pediatric use are as a medical countermeasure against anthrax and plague."

> Children treated with LEVAQUIN® had a significantly higher incidence of musculoskeletal disorders when compared to non-fluoroquinolone-treated children.

From April 2011 to March 2014, " <1% of total patients receiving a dispensed prescription for levofloxacin from US outpatient retail pharmacies were aged 0–16 years old." Source: Department of Health and Human Services Public Health Service Food and Drug Administration Center for Drug Evaluation and Research Office of Surveillance and Epidemiology Pediatric Post-marketing Pharmacovigilance and Drug Utilization Review Date: August 14, 2014).

We identified 32 pediatric cases of levofloxacin-associated adverse events in the FAERS database received by the FDA from April 1, 2011, to March 31, 2014.

This review did not identify any unlabeled, drug-related safety concerns that are clearly causally related to levofloxacin.

Pediatric death cases are confounded by patients who were administered levofloxacin to treat life-threatening diseases (i.e., CNS tuberculosis and meningitis), as well as multiple uses of concomitant medications, making it challenging to assess the role of levofloxacin on the outcome of death. These patients were severely ill prior to receiving the first dose of levofloxacin.

Pediatric patients aged 0–16 years old accounted for less than 1% (nearly 69,000 patients) of the total 17.6 million patients who received a dispensed prescription for oral levofloxacin tablets from U.S. outpatient retail pharmacies during the cumulative time period from April 2011 through March 2014. In the same time period, pediatric patients aged 0–16 years old accounted for 30% (nearly 9,900 patients) of the total 32,000 patients who received a dispensed prescription for oral levofloxacin solution from U.S. outpatient retail pharmacies. In the same time period, pediatric patients aged 0–16 years old accounted for less than 1% (nearly 19,000 patients) of the total 6.6 million patients who had a hospital billing for injectable levofloxacin from U.S. nonfederal hospitals (inpatient and outpatient ER).

No new safety concerns in pediatric patients were identified in this review of FAERS post-marketing reports of levofloxacin.

1.1.24 2014 FDA Dear Healthcare Professional Letters

In 2014, the FDA issued a guidance on Dear Healthcare Professional Letters. (FDA Guidance for Industry 2014). These letters communicate the highest level of concern by a manufacturer to providers related to safety and efficacy of a drug. They have become an important part of FDA's and manufacturers' approaches to ensuring FQ safety. As described by the FDA "This guidance provides recommendations to industry and FDA staff on the content and format of Dear Health Care Provider (DHCP) letters. DHCP letters are correspondence—often in the form of a mass mailing from the manufacturer or distributor of a human drug or biologic or from FDA—intended to alert physicians and other health care providers about important new or updated information regarding a human drug or biologic." The FDA notes that "DHCP letters may also be distributed by email and are often made available on the Internet (e.g., on company Web sites or through patient advocacy groups)." Under this Guidance, "Important Drug Warning letters" are described as being used to convey important new safety information that "concerns a significant hazard to health," as outlined in 21 CFR 200.5(c) [1]. This safety information could affect the decision to use a drug or require a change in behavior concerning the use of the drug, such as a specific type of monitoring.

This type of Dear Healthcare Professional letter is used to convey information that is being incorporated into one or more of the following sections of the prescribing information: "BOXED WARNINGS (Contains Nonbinding Recommendations); WARNINGS, CONTRAINDICATIONS, or WARNINGS AND PRECAUTIONS SECTIONS. Examples of the types of safety concerns that are communicated in Important Drug Warning letters include Previously unknown serious or life-threatening adverse reactions; clinically important new information about a known adverse reaction; identification of a subpopulation at greater risk in whom the drug should be used with added caution…; identification of a subpopulation in which the drug is contraindicated; a drug interaction or medication error that may result in a serious or life-threatening adverse reaction; implementation of a new or modified Risk Evaluation and Mitigation System (REMS)."

These "Important Drug Warnings" became an integral component to warning healthcare providers about serious ADRs associated with ciprofloxacin, but not for levofloxacin (see below).

1.1.25 2014 Citizen Petition

In September 2014, Drs. Bennett and Martin submitted a Citizen Petition to the FDA requesting that more warnings of psychiatric adverse events be added to the Levaquin label. The petition also asked the FDA to add a specific "Psychiatric Effects" heading on the Levaquin label which would include the following adverse events: toxic psychoses, restlessness, anxiety, confusion, hallucinations, paranoia, depression, nightmares, insomnia, suicidal thoughts or acts, feeling abnormal, loss of consciousness, disorientation, agitation, delirium, depressed level of consciousness, amnesia, coma, disturbance in attention, panic attack, memory impairment, and nervousness, noting that these events may start during treatment or may be delayed and start days, weeks, or months after the last dose. Finally, the petition requested that the FDA add psychiatric adverse events, including suicide, to the Levaquin Black Box, the most serious type of warning.

1.1.26 2014 Meeting with U.S. Senate Health Committee

In November 2014, Drs. Bennett and Martin met with staff from the U.S. Senate Health Committee, asking for the committee's assistance in asking the FDA to add more safety warnings to FQ labels.

1.1.27 2015 Meeting with FDA

In August 2015, Drs. Bennett and Martin and several "floxed" individuals participated in a meeting with FDA staff regarding FQ adverse events and FQ safety concerns.

1.1.28 2015 FQ Case Studies

In 2015, four case reports of Fluoroquinolone-associated neuropathy case series were published in BMJ Open report by Golomb et al. [Golomb]. The study reported a case series of four previously healthy, employed adults without significant prior medical history in each of whom symptoms developed while on FQs, with progression that continued the following discontinuation evolving to a severe, disabling multisymptomatic profile variably involving tendinopathy, muscle weakness, peripheral neuropathy, autonomic dysfunction, sleep disorder, cognitive dysfunction, and psychiatric disturbance. The authors advised that physicians and patients should be alert to the potential for FQ-induced severe disabling multi-symptom pathology that may persist and progress following FQ use. Known induction by FQs of delayed mitochondrial toxicity provides a compatible mechanism, with symptom profiles (and documented mechanisms of FQ toxicity) compatible with the hypothesis of an exposure-induced mitochondrial neurogastrointestinal encephalomyopathy.

1.1.29 2015 FDA Advisory Committee Meeting

On November 5, 2015, Dr. Bennett attended the FDA Joint Advisory Committee for Antibiotics and Drug Safety in Maryland and discussed FQ safety issues. At this meeting, FDA Epidemiologist Debra Boxwell, Ph.D. described the constellation of FQ adverse events as "Fluoroquinolone-Associated Disability (FQAD)" and defined it as disability which results in a "substantial disruption of a person's ability to conduct normal life functions" and having "adverse events reported from two or more of the following body systems: musculoskeletal, neuropsychiatric, peripheral nervous system, senses (vision, hearing, etc.), skin, cardiovascular". Deborah Boxwell further indicated that in order to meet this FQAD definition, these adverse events must "last 30 days or longer after stopping the fluoroquinolone."

Part of the meeting included the review of a literature review by Etian of the FDA on FQ and neurotoxicity and FQAD. The literature search identified two studies of FQs-associated peripheral neuropathy. The first study noted that peripheral neuropathy is an identified risk of systemic antibacterial therapy with FQs. The risk and its severity, including the development of Guillain-Barré syndrome between individual agents are uncertain. The study examined associations between FQs and peripheral neuropathy and Guillen-Barré Syndrome in cases spontaneously reported to the FDA Adverse Event Reporting System between 1997 and 2012. The Medical Dictionary for Regulatory Activities Preferred Term was used to define peripheral neuropathy and Guillen-Barré Syndrome. Individual FQs were identified by generic names and routes of administration. Empirical Bayes Geometric Mean (EBGM) with 95% confidence interval (EB05-EB95) was calculated as disproportionality measure. Safety signals with EB05 2 or more were considered significant disproportional increases in event reporting at least twice the times higher than that expected. Overall, 539 peripheral neuropathy reports out of 46,257 adverse event reports were submitted for FQs. Nine percent of peripheral neuropathy reports were for Guillen-Barré Syndrome. Significant disproportionality of peripheral neuropathy (EBGM 2.70; EB05–EB95 2.51–2.90) and Guillen-Barré Syndrome (EBGM 3.22; EB05–EB95 2.55–4.02) was identified for fluoroquinolones. Signals of peripheral neuropathy were detected for ciprofloxacin (EBGM 3.24; EB05–EB95 2.87–3.66) and levofloxacin (EBGM 3.36; EB05–EB95 3.02–3.72). A GBS signal was detected for ciprofloxacin (EBGM 4.15; EB05–EB95 2.94–5.74). Guillen-Barré Syndrome and Peripheral Neuropathy, respectively, ranked sixth and eighth among reported neurologic events. This study reinforced the link between FQs and peripheral neuropathy and showed the potential association with more severe forms of nerve damage.

At the November 2015 Advisory Committee meeting, FDA also reported an update on benefits and risk review of FQs. The FDA reviewed placebo-controlled clinical trials of various antibacterial drugs conducted in patients that have acute bacterial sinusitis (ABS), acute bacterial exacerbation of chronic bronchitis (ABECB), and uncomplicated urinary tract infections (UTI). Many of the trials were conducted from 2010 to 2015 years and some ABS and ABECB trials did not show a benefit over placebo. Some trials showed a treatment benefit for ABS and ABECB, and most trials showed a treatment benefit for uncomplicated UTI, but many patients who received a placebo had clinical resolution of their infection.

FDA also reported at the 2015 Advisory Committee meeting results of an updated review of adverse reactions associated with fluoroquinolone antibacterial drugs in order to re-evaluate risks and benefits of FQ antibacterial drugs for the treatment of these conditions. This review was of the FDA Adverse Event Reporting System (FAERS) database for reports logged in from November 1997 to May 2015. This review identified 178 U.S. cases of apparently healthy patients who took an oral fluoroquinolone to treat ABS, ABECB, or uncomplicated UTIs and developed disabling and potentially irreversible adverse reactions that appeared as a constellation of symptoms. Because it was difficult to clearly ascertain whether the report was for treatment of two of these indications, ABECB or uncomplicated UTI, the search was broadened to include the indications "bronchitis" and "urinary tract infections" in addition to ABS, ABECB, and uncomplicated UTI. Only patients who reported adverse reactions lasting longer than a month and involving two or more body systems (e.g., musculoskeletal, peripheral nervous system, neuropsychiatric, senses, cardiovascular, and skin) were included in the evaluation. The majority of the adverse reactions primarily affected the musculoskeletal system, peripheral nervous system, and central nervous system. The majority of cases (74%) were in patients 30–59 years. Many patients described how seriously the disability impacted their lives, including job loss and the resulting lack of health insurance, large medical bills, financial problems, and family tension or dissolution. The mean duration of the disabling adverse reactions at the time the report was received by FDA was 14 months, with the longest duration reported 9 years. Several cases reported that selected adverse reactions either resolved or improved; other cases reported that the reactions got worse or continued. It is possible these adverse reactions may be permanent. Long-term pain of any kind was the most commonly reported symptom, with 97% of all cases reporting pain associated with musculoskeletal adverse reactions. The ongoing neuropsychiatric adverse reactions were reported to be distressing, affecting employment and quality of life.

1.1.30   2015 FDA Listening Session

In 2015, the FDA conducted a listening session on FQ toxicities. The session occurred on April 23, 2015 and included four persons from a social network called "the Floxed Network" who reported personal experiences and a summary of concerns. It supported SONAR's 2014 Citizen Petition request for the addition of "possible mitochondrial toxicity" to the levofloxacin label. The FDA had received had 96 comments on the mitochondrial toxicity request.

1.1.31   2016 FQ Neuropsychiatric Study

In February 2016, SONAR and Drs. Bennett and Martin collaboratively published "Fluoroquinolone-related neuropsychiatric and mitochondrial toxicity: a collaborative investigation by scientists and members of a social network," by Kaur, et.al. [Ref: https://www.ncbi.nlm.nih.gov/pubmed/26955658] This study documents that "mice treated with ciprofloxacin had lower grip strengths, reduced balance, and depressive behavior compared with the controls." Additionally, this study describes that a survey of floxed individuals indicated that "93 of 94 respondents reported FQ-associated events including anxiety, depression, insomnia, panic attacks, clouded thinking, depersonalization, suicidal thoughts, psychosis, nightmares, and impaired memory beginning within days of FQ initiation or days to months of FQ discontinuation." Furthermore, this study concludes that "levofloxacin and ciprofloxacin toxicities were neurologic (30% and 26%, respectively), tendon damage (8 and 6%), and psychiatric (10 and 2%)."

1.1.32   2016 FQ Label Updates

On July 26, 2016, almost nine months after the November 2015 Advisory Committee meeting, the FDA requested that FQ manufacturers update the FQ product labels to disclose that FQs "have been associated with disabling and potentially irreversible serious adverse reactions that have occurred together, including tendinitis and tendon rupture, peripheral neuropathy, central nervous system effects." The FDA, however, failed to require FQ makers to warn of FQAD, as defined by FDA epidemiologist Dr. Boxwell, almost nine months earlier.

1.1.33   2016 FDA Response to Citizen Petition

It wasn't until July 2018, almost 4 years after Drs. Bennett and Martin submitted the Citizen Petition to the FDA, that the FDA approved the requests to require FQ manufacturers add additional psychiatric adverse events to the Levaquin label and to create a separate label subheading for psychiatric adverse events. This change would mean that often devastating psychiatric effects would no longer be meshed under the general central nervous system heading. Additionally, the FDA acknowledged that psychiatric adverse events, including suicide, were assumed to already be included in the Levaquin Black Box warning, as part of central nervous system events. Unfortunately, the FDA failed to acknowledge that most physicians and patients will not assume that central nervous system events include psychiatric side effects, including suicide. Because FQs have class effect, these label changes were applied to all FQs.

Because suicide is such a significant, under-recognized FQ adverse event, in September 2018 SONAR, Drs. Bennett and Martin and the SONAR team collaboratively reported "Fluoroquinolone-Associated Suicide," by Kommalapati, et al. https://www.ncbi.nlm.nih.gov/pubmed/30031596. This study describes that "several case reports have raised concerns that exposure to fluoroquinolones (FQs) may increase the risk of suicidal behavior." This study explains that "of the 122 FQ-associated suicide or suicide-attempt events reported to the FDA, 108 met inclusion criteria" for the study, and "half of the events described completed suicides." It further describes that "40% of the events occurred within two weeks of FQ initiation." Finally, this study "highlights the importance of continued awareness of FQ-associated suicide-related events, which can occur even in patients without prior psychiatric illness."

1.1.34   2018 FQ Nature Article

In March 2018, Dr. Bennett and the collaborative work with Dr. Martin, SONAR, and Andrew Bennett, an undergraduate at the University of South Carolina, were featured in a three-page Nature article, "When antibiotics turn toxic," by Jo Marchant. In this article, Dr. Bennett explains that "prior work (from his National Institutes of Health-funded research) found that only 1% of serious adverse events associated with four commonly used drugs were reported to the FDA, suggesting that fluoroquinolones might have harmed hundreds of thousands of people in the United States alone". The Nature article also discusses findings reported by Andrew Bennett at a national oncology meeting regarding a gene identified that appears to be associated with increased risk for ciprofloxacin-associated neuropsychiatric toxicity.

1.1.35   2019 Citizen Petition

In October 2019, Drs. Bennett and Martin submitted another Citizen Petition to the FDA, this time asking for warnings of FQAD to be added to the Levaquin label, asking for psychiatric adverse events to be specifically identified in the Black Box warnings, and asking for a Levaquin Risk Evaluation and Mitigation Strategy (REMS) which would require patients to give written consent prior to taking Levaquin.

1.1.36   2019 FQ Neuropsychiatric Toxicity Study

In November 2019, SONAR, Andrew Bennett, and Drs. Bennett and Martin published "An evaluation of reports of ciprofloxacin, levofloxacin, and moxifloxacin-association neuropsychiatric toxicities, long-term disability, and aortic aneurysms/dissections disseminated by the Food and Drug Administration and the European Medicines Agency." This study notes that the FDA and the European Medicines Agency "report that neuropsychiatric toxicity, long-term disability, and aortic dissections/aneurysms occur with all FQs. Disability and neuropsychiatric toxicity can occur after one dose or several months after FQs. United States' and European' regulators warn physicians not to prescribe FQs for uncomplicated acute urinary tract infection, sinusitis, or bronchitis, unless other possible choices are tried first, as risks outweigh benefits in these settings."

1.2   Discussion

As described in the October 2011 FDA "Guidance for Industry, Warnings and Precautions, Contraindications, and Boxed Warning Sections of Labeling" document: "A boxed warning is ordinarily used to highlight for prescribers … an adverse reaction so serious in proportion to the potential benefit from the drug … that it is essential that it be considered in assessing the risks and benefits of using the drug" of if "there is a serious adverse reaction that can be prevented or reduced in frequency or severity …".[3]

Consistent with this FDA Guidance regarding when to add a boxed warning to a drug label, FQAD clearly meets the FDA requirement that the adverse reaction—or in this case the "constellation of disabling symptoms"—are so serious that the FDA has included the word "Disabling" in its name. Furthermore, by the FDA's definition of FQAD, this constellation of symptoms may continue well past the discontinuation of taking the medication and may disrupt "a person's ability to conduct normal life functions."

1.3   Conclusions

1. The FDA had an unacceptably slow response to warn of the dangers of FQs.
2. Many people have needlessly died or have been needlessly, severely disabled following the use of FQs without adequate safety warnings.
3. The FDA has failed to adequately warn physicians and patients about the dangers of these commonly prescribed antibiotics.

---

[3] https://www.fda.gov/regulatory-information/search-fda-guidancedocuments/ warnings-and-precautions-contraindications-and-boxed-warning-sections-labeling-humanprescription.

1.3.1   Recommendations

As defined in Chap. 9 of the Federal Food, Drug and Cosmetics Act, the FDA shall "protect the public health" by ensuring that human "drugs are safe". Based on the research and issues included in this study, the FDA should:

1. Take action to require FQ manufacturers to add FQAD to the FQ labels;
2. To specifically identify psychiatric adverse events, including suicide, in FQ boxed warnings; and
3. To implement an FQ Risk Evaluation and Mitigation Strategy (REMS).

The FDA should act now to adequately warn physicians and patients about the dangers of FQ antibiotics. For more than a decade, Drs. Bennett and Martin and others have worked tirelessly to disclose serious, disabling, often permanent FQ adverse events. Now, it is time for the FDA to act.

Based on the extensive psychiatric and neurological adverse events documented in the FAERS data, it is recommended an FQ Patient Compensation Fund, similar to the National Football League (NFL) Concussion Fund, be established, funded by the makers of FQ antibiotics, to compensate individuals who suffer disabling post-FQ psychiatric or neurological adverse events.

1.3.2   Significance of This FQ Study

This study further expands the understanding of FQ neurological and psychiatric adverse events by describing cases of individuals suffering from these adverse events who have had abnormal neurological or psychiatric test results. This appears to be the first study to examine specific abnormal neurological and psychiatric test results related to post-FQ consumption.

1.4   REMS Request

FDA's Guidance for REMS requires the FDA is to consider the following six statutory factors in its analysis:

1. *The seriousness of any known or potential adverse events that may be related to the drug and the background incidence of such events in the population likely to use the drug;*
2. *The expected benefit of the drug with respect to the disease or condition;*
3. *The seriousness of the disease or condition that is to be treated with the drug;*
4. *Whether the drug is a new molecular entity;*
5. *The expected or actual duration of treatment with the drug; and*
6. *The estimated size of the population likely to use the drug.*

See April 2019 "Guidance for Industry REMS: FDA's Application of Statutory Factors In Determining When a REMS Is Necessary" ("Guidance").

The following documents the grounds for the request to implement a new REMS for Levaquin:

1. *The seriousness of any known or potential adverse events that may be related to the drug and the background incidence of such events in the population likely to use the drug;*

a. The seriousness of any known or potential adverse events that may be related to the drug:

Levaquin FQAD and Psychiatric Adverse Events are serious, have a significant impact on quality of life, and may only be prevented or reduced if physicians and patients are properly educated and aware of the risk-benefit calculus through a REMS.

Levaquin Fluoroquinolone-Associated Disability (FQAD), a "constellation of disabling symptoms" which results in "a substantial disruption of a person's ability to conduct normal life functions," includes adverse events which "last 30 days or longer after stopping the fluoroquinolone," and including adverse events from two or more of the following body systems: musculoskeletal, neuropsychiatric, peripheral nervous system, senses (vision, hearing, etc.), skin, and cardiovascular," clearly do not outweigh the benefit when Levaquin is used for many FDA-approved purposes.

Levaquin Psychiatric Adverse Events, including, toxic psychoses, hallucinations, paranoia, suicidal thoughts or acts, loss of consciousness, delirium, depressed level of consciousness, amnesia, coma, and memory impairment are all serious in that the risk of experiencing these potentially life-threatening symptoms do not outweigh the benefit when Levaquin is used for many FDA-approved purposes.

b. The background incidence of such events in the population likely to use the drug:

From December 1996 to May 2016, the FDA Adverse Events Reporting System (FAERS) received:

- **28,079** Levaquin adverse event **individual reports**,
- identifying **110,292** Levaquin **adverse events**, and
- identifying **1,765** Levaquin **deaths**.

It is broadly assumed that only 1% to 10% of actual adverse events are reported to the FDA.

Because Levaquin lacked adequate adverse events warnings for a significant period of time during the period of December 1996–May 2016, as evidenced by the updated Levaquin label safety warnings in recent years, it is assumed that only 1% of Levaquin adverse events have been reported to the FDA.

Thus, from December 1996 to May 2016, it is estimated:

- The actual number of Levaquin adverse events individual reports is estimated to be 2,807,900.
- The actual number of Levaquin adverse events is estimated to be 11,029,200.
- The actual number of Levaquin deaths is estimated to be 176,500.

When the above data is adjusted to include Levaquin individuals reports, adverse events, and deaths for the past 3 years from May 2016 to May 2019, it is assumed that from December 1996 to May 2019:

- The actual number of Levaquin adverse events **individual reports** is estimated to be **3,239,885**.
- The actual number of Levaquin **adverse events** is estimated to be **12,726,000**.
- The actual number of Levaquin **deaths** is estimated to be **203,654**.

The FDA's own FAERS data documents the extensive adverse event and death risks associated with Levaquin.

2. *The expected benefit of the drug with respect to the disease or condition*

While Levaquin is documented to treat complicated and uncomplicated infections, there are other alternative antibiotics which are not associated with FQAD or disabling and potentially irreversible serious psychiatric adverse events, including suicide and suicide-associated events.

3. *The seriousness of the disease or condition that is to be treated with the drug*

Levaquin is approved by the FDA to treat both complicated and uncomplicated infections.

4. *Whether the drug is a new molecular entity*

Levaquin is not a new molecular entity.

5. *The expected or actual duration of treatment with the drug*

The duration of treatment with Levaquin varies and is identified by the FDA on the Levaquin label. Levaquin's disabling and potentially irreversible adverse events, including FQAD and psychiatric adverse events, including suicide and suicide-associated events may be, as stated by the FDA, "irreversible," thus lasting a lifetime after taking Levaquin has been discontinued.

6. *The estimated size of the population likely to use the drug*

In 2018, over 7,000,000 prescriptions were written for Levaquin and its generic equivalents each year. Cite new numbers?

Additionally, the FDA Guidance on when to offer a REMS includes other factors to consider, including (1) the reliability of scientific evidence of the adverse effect, (2) whether the adverse effect is irreversible, (3) the frequency, (4) the ability to avoid the risk of occurrence through mitigating factors, and (5) whether information about the risk is already well-spread.

(1) Reliability of Levaquin Research

FQAD and other adverse effects of Levaquin are well established by years of research. The research has already been relied on extensively by the FDA in the past to require label changes and black box warnings, as outlined above.[4]

(2) Levaquin Adverse Events May Be Irreversible

As indicated above, the current Levaquin Black Box warning describes that Levaquin is "associated with disabling and potentially irreversible serious adverse reactions…."

Importantly, there is NO treatment for FQAD.

(3) Frequency and Seriousness of Levaquin Adverse Events

As described above, when the FDA FAERS data is adjusted for Levaquin individuals reports, adverse events, and deaths, the following are Levaquin estimates from December 1996 to May 2019:

- The actual number of Levaquin adverse events **individual reports** is estimated to be **3,239,885**
- The actual number of Levaquin **adverse events** is estimated to be **12,726,000**
- The actual number of Levaquin **deaths** is estimated to be **203,654**.

The FDA's own FAERS data documents the extensive adverse event and death risks associated with Levaquin.

Regarding the seriousness of Levaquin adverse events, again, as indicated above, the current Levaquin Black Box warning describes that Levaquin is "associated with disabling and potentially irreversible serious adverse reactions…."

Again, and importantly, there is NO treatment for FQAD.

(4) Ability to Avoid Levaquin's Risks

Currently there is no way to administer Levaquin in a manner that would reduce the risk of FQAD, serious psychiatric adverse events, including suicide and suicide-related events, or other disabling and potentially irreversible serious adverse events.

Moreover, apart from patients that have previously experienced a harmful Levaquin side effect, there are currently no additional means of identifying patients who may be at increased risk.

Indeed, improved Levaquin Black Box warnings and the addition of a Levaquin REM represent the only ways to reduce risk.

---

[4] As recently as July of 2018 the FDA issued a warning about the mental health side effects of FQs. *See* FDA July 10, 2018 Announcement (Attachment 3).

(5) Current Availability of Levaquin Risk Information

The current labeling regime is incomplete, FQAD has not been included anywhere on the labeling and importantly, is not included in the Levaquin Black Box, despite the fact that the FDA identified this constellation of disabling symptoms as far back as 2013.

Levaquin REMS Request Summary

In sum, the all-important first factor identified in the FDA REMS Guidance to determine if a REMS is required is:

> A drug that is **associated with a risk of a serious adverse event that is irreversible**, such as one that causes a permanent disability or persistent incapacity, may be particularly likely to have a favorable benefit-risk profile only in the presence of a REMS that helps minimize drug exposure and the associated occurrence of the adverse event.) Guidance p. 6.

It is unequivocal that Levaquin meets this requirement in that the current Levaquin Black Box states that:

> **Fluoroquinolones, including LEVAQUIN®, have been "associated with disabling and potentially irreversible serious adverse reactions…"**

Since the FDA has already clearly stated in the Levaquin Black Box that Levaquin is **"associated with disabling and potentially irreversible serious adverse reactions…"** this indicates a Levaquin REMS is necessary and appropriate.

Moreover, the FDA REMS Guidance states that "[s]uch REMS are designed to ensure that patients are fully informed of the serious risk before beginning therapy and may involve patient acknowledgment forms or other methods of documenting that such patient-provider discussions have taken place. This kind of REMS is particularly important for drugs with limited available methods of preventing the actual occurrence of drug-associated adverse events."

As indicated above, there is NO method for preventing the actual occurrence of Levaquin-associated adverse events. This further indicates that a Levaquin REMS is necessary and appropriate.

In sum, FQAD and serious psychiatric adverse events, including suicide and suicide-related adverse events are frequent, widespread, may be irreversible, and cannot be prevented.

Therefore, Levaquin should be subject to a REMS that includes "prescriber decisions about treatment with the drug. Such REMS are designed to ensure that patients are fully informed of the serious risk before beginning therapy and may involve patient acknowledgment forms or other methods of documenting that such patient-provider discussions have taken place." See Guidance.

EVIDENCE REVIEW FOR FLUOROQUINOLONE-ASSOCIATED DIS-ABILITY (FQAD). 2001: Survey of persons with fluoroquinolone-associated neuropathy conducted by Jay Cohen MD. A survey of cases of fluoroquinolone-associated adverse events that included peripheral nervous system (PNS) symptoms was posted on Internet Web sites. Cases were obtained with the assistance of members of Web sites formed by people sustaining fluoroquinolone-related events. Information obtained met the standards of Med-Watch, and each reported case was assessed using the Naranjo probability scale. Overall, 36 of the 45 cases reported severe events that typically involved multiple organ systems. Symptoms had lasted more than three months in 71% of cases and more than one year in 58%. Onset of adverse events was usually rapid, with 15 (33%) events beginning within 24 hours of initiating treatment, 26 (58%) within 72 hours, and 38 (84%) within one week. Sixty courses of fluoroquinolones were prescribed: levofloxacin (n = 33 cases), ciprofloxacin ($n = 11$), ofloxacin ($n = 6$), lomefloxacin ($n = 1$), trovafloxacin ($n = 1$); in eight cases the same antibiotic was prescribed twice. The survey suggested a possible association between fluoro-quinolone antibiotics and severe, long-term adverse effects involving the peripheral nervous system and other organ systems. The severity of these cases may reflect a different population than typically reported to drug companies or to the FDA, which often originate from healthcare providers. The survey is the first paper to document the wide range of symptoms observed in persons with levofloxacin-associated neurologic toxicity. Cohen JS. Peripheral neuropathy associated with fluoro-quinolones. Ann Pharmacother. 2001 Dec;35(12):1540–7. doi: 10.1345/aph.1Z429. PMID: 11793615. 2001 FDA Office of Surveillance and Epidemiology Review. This review was the result of a patient contacting the FDA. agency. The review (Singer, Sally. Office of Safety and Epidemiology (OSE) Post-marketing Safety Review: Peripheral Neuropathy with Levofloxacin. 30 Apr 2001), identified 28 cases of peripheral neuropathy associated with levofloxacin use. It found that peripheral neuropathy lasted as long as two years after patients received levo-floxacin. 2003-FDA Second Review on Neuropathy conducted by the Office of Surveillance and Epidemiology. This review, completed in 2003 (Singer, Sally. OSE Post-marketing Safety Review: Prolonged Peripheral Neuropathies with Flu-oroquinolones. 06 June 2003), described 108 cases of peripheral neuropathy associated with ciprofloxacin, levofloxacin, and/or ofloxacin use. Thirty-four of the 108 cases reported peripheral neuropathy at time periods of a year or more after the drug had been discontinued, suggesting potential irreversibility of the condition. The review recommended that peripheral neuropathy be added to the labeling for ciprofloxacin and levofloxacin. 2010; In 2010, toxicologist Yvonne Will (senior author) and her colleagues at Pfizer in Groton, Connecticut, reported an assay to detect mitochondrial damage early in drug development. They found that some antibiotics affected mitochondria and others didn't. Every fluoroquinolone they tested damaged mitochondria in human liver cells—having what the researchers described as "a strong effect" at therapeutic concentrations, although Will cautions that it isn't possible to extrapolate from that result to clinical outcomes. Reference: Nadanaciva S, Dillman K, Gebhard DF, Shrikhande A, Will Y. High-content screening for compounds that affect mtDNA-encoded protein levels in eukaryotic cells. J Biomol Screen. 2010 Sep;15(8):937–48. doi: 10.1177/1087057110373547. Epub 2010 Jul 12. 2013: PubMed Literature search on Levaquin-associated neu-ropathy conducted by FDA

References

1. Bhanu MU, Kondapi AK (2010) Neurotoxic activity of a topoisomerase-I inhibitor, camptothecin, in cultured cerebellar granule neurons. Neurotoxicology 31:730–737
2. Champoux JJ (2001) DNA topoisomerases: structure, function, and mechanism. Ann Rev Biochem 70:369–413
3. Fang C et al (2012) Oxidative stress inhibits sexual transport: implications for neurodegenerative diseases. Mol Neurodegener 7:29
4. Freeman MZ et al (2021) Fluoroquinolones-associated disability: it is not all in your head. NeuroSci 2(3):235–253. https://doi.org/10.3390/neurosci2030017
5. Golomb BA, Koslik HJ, Redd AJ (2015) Fluoroquinolone-induced serious, persistent, multisymptomatic adverse effects. BMJ Case Rep 5:2015:bcr2015209821
6. Hulgan T et al (2005) Mitochondrial haplogroups and peripheral neuropathy dur antiretroviral therapy. AIDS 19:1341–1349
7. Kabbani S et al (2018) Opportunities to improve fluoroquinolone prescribing in the united states for adult ambulatory care visits. Clin Infect Dis Off Publ Infect Dis Soc Am 67:134–136
8. Kohler JJ, Lewis W (2007) A brief overview of mechanisms of mitochondrial toxicity from NRTIs. Environ Mol Mutagen 48:166–172
9. Kondapi AK, Mulpuri N, Mandraju RK et al (2004) Analysis of age dependent changes of topoisomerase II α and β in rate brain. Int J Devl Neuroscience 22:19–30

Charles L. Bennett MD, Ph.D., MPP, SmartState Chair and Frank P. and Josie M. Fletcher Chair of Medication Safety and Efficacy and Director, SmartState Center for Medication Safety and Efficacy, is also a Visiting Scholar at the City of Hope National Cancer Institute Designated Comprehensive Cancer Center in Duarte, California and is the co-editor of this book, Cancer Policy (2nd Edition). Dr. Bennett is a Phi Beta Kappa and High Honors graduate in mathematics from Swarthmore College, earned his medical degree in 1981 from the University of Pennsylvania Perelman School of Medicine, and completed internal medicine, hematology, and oncology training at the Michael Reese Hospital and the University of Chicago Pritzger School of Medicine before completing his Ph.D. and Masters In Public Policy degrees with honors in social science at the RAND Pardee Graduate School of Public Policy in Santa Monica, California. He has led a 20-year National Institutes of Health funded pharmacovigilance called the Research on Adverse Drug events And Reports (RADAR) and subsequently called to Southern Network on Adverse drug Reactions (SONAR) at the University of South Carolina College of Pharmacy.

Oscar Champigneulle is a junior at Brown University in Providence, Rhode Island. During a semester that was interrupted by absence of in-person classes due to the COVID-19 pandemic, he conducted investigations of pharmaceutical safety. His two foci were hematologic complications of COVID-19 vaccinations and disability-related complications following fluroquinolone administration.

Andrew Bennett BA is a graduate of the University of South Carolina Honors Program with a Magna Cum Laude award. He was funded in part by grants from the American Cancer Society Institutional Research Grant Award and the University of South Carolina's Science Undergraduate Research Fellowship under the leadership of Zaina Qureshi, Ph.D. and Carolyn Bannister, Ph.D. to investigate genetic risk factors for fluoroquinolone-associated disability. The initial work was presented in 2017 at the Association of Veteran's Administration Hematology and Oncology conference in Denver and covered in more detail in Nature in a news article by Jo Marchant "When antibiotics turn toxic: commonly prescribed drugs called fluoroquinolones cause rare, disturbing side effects. Researchers are struggling to work out why." (March 7, 2018; 555: 431–438). He will begin post-graduate studies focusing on quinolone-associated toxicity at Oxford University in England in October 2021.

Bartlett Witherspoon MBA is a third-year medical student at the Medical University of South Carolina and a graduate of Vanderbilt University's Master's in Business Administration program. He is an active co-investigator with Dr. Bennett and the SONAR project and has been a lead co-investigator on published manuscripts on fluoroquinolone-associated disability and on biosimilar oncology products.

Cecilia Bove Ph.D. graduated with a Bachelor's Degree in Biotechnology and a Master's Degree in Medical Biotechnology from the University of Perugia, Perugia, Italy. She then studied the involvement of the vagus nerve in Parkinson's Disease at Penn State College of Medicine, Hershey, Pennsylvania, where she obtained a Ph.D. in Neuroscience in 2019. Dr. Bove is currently a Visiting Assistant Professor in Neurobiology at Bucknell University, Lewisburg, Pennsylvania, where she is investigating how Fluoroquinolones antibiotics may negatively impact gastrointestinal function.

Biosimilar Epoetin in the United States: A View from the Southern Network on Adverse Reactions

Sumimasa Nagai, Bartlett Witherspoon, Chadi Nabhan, and Charles L. Bennett

2.1 Introduction

Biosimilar drugs, close copies of patented biologicals, are intended to provide access to less expensive, highly similar versions of reference (previously approved) biological agents [1]. The biological epoetin accounts for $1.8 billion in drug spending annually worldwide (primarily for the treatment of anemia due to chronic kidney disease or anemia due to cancer chemotherapy).

Mature epoetin biosimilar markets exist in the European Union (EU) countries since 2007 and in Japan since 2010, as five epoetin biosimilar formulations have received regulatory authorizations in the EU countries and one in Japan, respectively [2, 3]. Biosimilar epoetins now account for most of the EU epoetin sales (varying by country) and also most of the epoetin sales in Japan [2–4].

Herein, we review information on epoetin biosimilar reviewed by the FDA Oncologic Drugs Advisory Committee (ODAC) in May 2017, the concerns and conclusions expressed by ODAC, and related topics of regulation, litigation, interchangeability, substitution, naming, and labeling that will affect the uptake of this product upon licensing for use in the United States. SONAR also reviewed the current status of biosimilar epoetins in the United States. Search strategy and selection criteria. We reviewed relevant peer-reviewed articles with the use of MEDLINE (PubMed), Embase (Ovid), and Web of Science. Search terms included: "filgrastim," "biosimilars", "follow-on biologics", "similar biologic products", "subsequent entry biologics", "follow-on biologic products", and "similar biologic medicinal products". The search was restricted to papers published between January

S. Nagai · B. Witherspoon · C. Nabhan · C. L. Bennett (✉)
SONAR (Southern Network on Adverse Reactions) Program, University of South Carolina College of Pharmacy, Columbia, SC 29208, USA
e-mail: bennettc@cop.sc.edu

S. Nagai
e-mail: sunagai@kuhp.kyoto-u.ac.jp

2005 and January 2017, in English or Japanese, and either comments, editorials, journal articles, reviews, or systematic reviews addressing biosimilar filgrastims in Japan and/or the United States. Additional non-peer-reviewed literature was included in this Policy Review and identified through a Google search and from citations in several key articles.

2.1.1 Regulatory Approval for Epoetin Biosimilar in the United States

The Biologic Price Competition and Innovation Act of 2009 created an abbreviated biosimilar licensure pathway. These 351(k) regulations require demonstrating a high degree of "similarity" of biosimilar with reference epoetin—comparing physicochemical and immunochemical properties, biological activity, specifications, stability, safety, and efficacy [1]. The "totality of the evidence" supports regulatory approval [1]. The step-wise approach characterizes residual uncertainty at each step. The rationale is that a biosimilar shown to be analytically and functionally similar to a reference biologic will behave like the reference biologic clinically. This approach begins with a demonstration of structural and functional characterization of the proposed biosimilar and the reference biologic. Once analytical similarity is demonstrated, an assessment is made of the amount of residual uncertainty with respect to structure/function characterization and the potential for clinically meaningful differences. In contrast to the EU requirements, FDA requires animal in vivo studies and that the reference biosimilar is a US-approved product.

In May 2017, The Oncology Drug Advisory Committee of the Food and Drug Administration reviewed the application of Hospira epoetin biosimilar and recommended regulatory approval from the FDA for the same clinical indications as the reference biologic (epoetin, manufactured by Amgen).

2.1.2 Chemistry, Manufacturing, and Controls

Endogenous erythropoietin (EPO), produced mainly by the kidney, stimulates erythropoiesis. EPO binds to EPO receptors on lineage-committed erythroid progenitor cells, initiating signal transduction that results in proliferation and differentiation into red blood cells. Pharmacodynamic (PD) measures include reticulocyte count and serum hemoglobin levels. Epoetin alfa is a 165 amino acid recombinant protein that has the same amino acid sequence as endogenous erythropoietin.

The epoetin biosimilar product was compared to reference epoetin with physicochemical and functional methods. Amino acid sequences of the products were shown to be the same. Glycosylation, a post-translational modification necessary for protein function and stability, was shown to occur at the same arginine and serine-residue sites. However, the composition of the glycans is complex, varies among different EPO products, and is attributed to manufacturing process differences. This glycosylation contributes to the pharmacokinetics (PK) of endogenous and recombinant EPO, mainly by increasing EPO's half-life. Residual differences were noted in glycosylation.

The proposed epoetin biosimilar is produced in Chinese Hamster Ovary cells transfected with the human EPO gene. The manufacturing process consists of steps intended to isolate and purify EPO. The sponsors demonstrated that process-related impurities including host cell proteins, host cell DNA, and host retrovirus-like particles were reduced to low levels in the manufacturing process. The product was developed as a liquid injection in single-use vials at the same strengths as approved for reference epoetin.

Formulations of the products differed with respect to inactive ingredients and pH. The material used in non-clinical studies was manufactured using processes that differed from the final commercial process with respect to EPO content. Data presented at the meeting indicated that these differences did not affect safety assessments and conclusions of non-clinical studies. FDA reviewers agreed that the biosimilar epoetin manufacturing processes were valid, produced products of consistent quality, and that formulation differences did not have clinical effects.

Analytical similarity data were provided by the applicant. An independent analysis of these data and associated statistical analyses were reported by FDA reviewers. When differences occurred, FDA reviewers indicated that they assessed these differences based on publicly available data and evaluated whether the applicant had an adequate control strategy in place to evaluate the attributes. Reference epoetin contains human serum albumin at concentrations that interfered with analytical analysis. The sponsor developed procedures for removing human serum albumin to facilitate analytical comparisons in settings where this did not impact specific quality attributes. These studies evaluated primary structure, glycosylation, higher-order structure, biological activity, drug product attributes, and product-related substances and impurities. Minor structural differences were noted.

Mean EPO content of the proposed epoetin biosimilar was demonstrated by the applicant as being within the biological activity range of reference epoetin. FDA reviewers' independent analysis of the applicant's data agreed. Of note, the 2015 marketing application of a biosimilar epoetin from the same sponsor, using a different commercial process, found a 3.5% difference in mean EPO content. This difference was attributed to a resolvable manufacturing issue, successfully addressed after the 2015 submission.

2.1.3   Biological Activity

Biological activity was evaluated using assays directed to the mechanism of action, focusing on EPO receptor binding, cell proliferation induction, and reticulocyte production. Tests included a competitive receptor-binding ELISA assay, surface plasmon resonance measurement, an *in vitro* cell-based bioassay using a human leukemic cell line (UT-7), and a compendial-based in vivo normothymic mouse assay (mice reticulocyte production was measured). Statistical equivalence analyses for in vitro and in vivo studies were assessed by FDA reviewers as being within the acceptance criteria and within the accepted quality range defined based on the reference biologic. FDA reviewers concluded that these data supported a conclusion of biosimilar biological activity and that glycosylation differences did not result in observable differences in mouse biological activity. Seven comparisons of the type and levels of product-related substances and product impurities supported a conclusion of high biosimilarity. Biosimilarity was also demonstrated for subvisible particles, which are implicated as potential causes of anti-product antibodies using microflow imaging and nanoparticle tracking analyses.

2.1.4 Pharmacology/Toxicology

The two products were compared in two head-to-head studies assessing PD, PK, and toxicity in rats and dogs. Some comparisons could be evaluated only in Beagle dogs with intravenous epoetin administration. The sponsor and the FDA concluded that, while residual uncertainties exist in the two products based on non-clinical data, these differences did not observably affect PK/PD similarity and comparative clinical studies. The sponsor and FDA reviewers noted that recombinant epoetin protein is not species-specific and therefore animal toxicology studies were relevant to predicting potential human effects. Again, the sponsor and FDA reviewers concluded that residual uncertainties existed in the PK/PD studies of the biosimilar in rats and dogs and needed to be addressed in PK/PD studies in human and in comparative clinical studies.

2.1.5 Immunogenicity

This aspect of the submission was extensively discussed and reviewed. Studies in 2000 and in 2004 identified clinically significant cases of anti-erythropoietin antibody-mediated pure red cell aplasia (PRCA) with subcutaneous administration of the Eprex formulation of epoetin. In 2010, two cases of anti-erythropoietin antibody-mediated PRCA had been identified with subcutaneous administration of the proposed biosimilar during the conduct of a phase III trial among chronic kidney disease (CKD) patients. Root cause analyses identified tungsten leaching from syringe pins and manufacturing process changes fixed this problem. The incidence of immunogenicity for the two products was compared in 3 multiple-dose, parallel-arm studies of 849 patients with CKD and 129 healthy volunteers. No neutralizing antidrug antibodies were identified, and no apparent impact of anti-drug antibodies on safety, PK, or PD endpoints were observed.

2.1.6 Clinical Pharmacology

The sponsor submitted to the FDA one randomized open-label cross-over study in 81 healthy subjects that compared PK, PD, safety, and tolerability of a single 100

U/kilogram subcutaneous dose of the 2 products and 1 randomized open-label parallel-group study of 129 healthy subjects receiving 100 U/kilogram three times per week subcutaneously. The results were interpreted by the applicant and FDA reviewers as supporting conclusions of no clinically meaningful differences in PK and PD between products.

2.1.7 Clinical Efficacy and Safety

The sponsor also submitted to the FDA two randomized, double-blinded, parallel-group clinical trials that enrolled patients with chronic kidney disease on hemodialysis who were receiving epoetin maintenance treatment with co-primary endpoints of differences between arms in mean weekly hemoglobin levels and mean weekly dose. One study evaluated 246 patients who received subcutaneous drug one to three times per week. The other study evaluated 612 patients who received intravenous drug three times per week. Safety assessments did not identify significant differences between products. The efficacy analyses reported that 90% confidence intervals for the outcome values were within pre-determined equivalence margins.

2.1.8 Risk Evaluation and Mitigations Strategy (REMS)

FDA reviewers noted that the 2010 requirement for a REMS program for ESAs in the oncology setting had ended in April 2017 as the FDA determined that it was no longer needed to ensure that the benefits of ESAs outweighed risks. The sponsor's proposed product labeling and medication guide, similar to that of reference epoetin, identify increased risks of tumor progression or recurrence, death, myocardial infarction, stroke, venous thromboembolism, and thrombosis of vascular access.

2.1.9 Extrapolation

The sponsor requested FDA licensure for all indications for which the reference epoetin is licensed. These included: anemia treatment for patients with CKD, including patients not on dialysis or who are receiving dialysis; for treatment of anemia due to zidovudine; for treatment of chemotherapy-induced anemia (CIA) among persons with non-myeloid malignancies; and to reduce the need for allogeneic red blood cell transfusions among patients who are at high risk for peri-operative blood loss from elective non-cardiac, non-vascular surgery. FDA reviewers indicated that the mechanism of action of epoetin is the same as endogenous EPO, biosimilar epoetin is highly similar to reference epoetin, PK/PD was similar in healthy subjects, and similar efficacy between the two products was demonstrated in animals; the frequency of anti-drug antibodies with the proposed biosimilar was low in clinical studies programs evaluating healthy subjects and

CKD patients; and similar clinical safety and clinical efficacy was demonstrated between the products among patients with CKD on hemodialysis. While biosimilarity was tested clinically only among CKD patients, FDA reviewers concluded that the evidence supported the sponsor's request for extrapolation for use in approved indications for reference epoetin.

2.1.10 Findings of the Oncology Drug Advisory Committee (ODAC) of the FDA

In 2017, ODAC advisors voted 14 to 1 in favor of recommending the sponsor's biosimilar epoetin application for FDA approval of five dosages of single-unit vials corresponding to FDA-approved dosages of reference epoetin for subcutaneous administration. ODAC reviewers were supportive of analytical comparability findings and that there were no detectable clinically meaningful differences. Some panelists expressed concerns about whether data surrounding immunogenicity could be extrapolated to support approval for all indications. One panelist voted against approving the application, noting that he did not support approval for two indications because of a lack of data on immunogenicity and safety in these settings. The other 14 panelists agreed that residual uncertainty related to immunogenicity and extrapolation for all indications existed, but a clearer picture would emerge with post-marketing surveillance. Subsequently, the FDA did not approve this epoetin biosimilar formulation, primarily due to manufacturing quality concerns identified at five of the manufacturer's plants worldwide. Following extensive quality changes at these plants, FDA approved the biosimilar epoetin formulation in 2018.

2.1.11 Patents and Litigation

The US epoetin primary patent expired in 2015. In an ongoing Federal Court case, Amgen has claimed that the biosimilar sponsor (Hospira) infringes two patents (US Patent Nos. 5,856,298 and 5,756,349). Subsequent litigation between Hospira and Amgen for biosimilar epoetin focuses on the "patent dance" a process that requires biosimilar sponsors to share information with the reference biologic sponsor in advance of FDA approval and, at the time of FDA approval to market, a 180-day notification of intent to market epoetin biosimilar is required. Amgen filed an appeal in Federal Court from a discovery order made in District Court litigation. The District Court had denied Amgen's motion to compel Hospira to produce certain documents regarding its proposed biosimilar, finding that the information sought was not relevant to patents asserted in the first wave litigation.

2.1.12   Naming and Labeling

Naming and labeling conventions are important because biosimilars and reference biologics do not have identical chemical characteristics, as noted above. FDA recently finalized Labeling and Naming Guidances [5, 6]. Product-specific suffixes are recommended as the best way to track specific biologics or biosimilars through the supply chain, to facilitate pharmacovigilance [5]. The Naming Guidance attaches random four-letter suffixes for reference and biosimilar epoetin and includes the same epoetin base name. The Labeling Guidance requires prominent inclusion of biosimilar information that supported approval and inclusion of a formal statement that the Hospira epoetin product is a biosimilar. Hospira must revise product labeling on an ongoing basis, without conditioning changes on reference epoetin labeling. The accepted name for the epoetin biosimilar is epoetin-epbx.

2.1.13   Interchangeability

The 2017 FDA Draft Biosimilar Interchangeability Guidance outlines proposed regulatory criteria for determining biosimilar interchangeable designations [7]. The sponsor of epoetin biosimilar did not request designation as an interchangeable, as this is a higher order regulatory request that has not been finalized by regulation.

2.1.14   Substitution

Substitution was discussed extensively at the 2017 ODAC meeting. To date, 37 states have passed legislation preventing substitution irrespective of biosimilars being deemed interchangeable [8]. In all states, the specific name of the epoetin product must be recorded. In some states, the prescribing physician must be contacted and recipient patients must be contacted or notified before epoetin substitution occurs. No clear path forward on substitution was recommended, realizing that this is a state pharmacy board and legislative issue.

2.1.15   Pharmacovigilance and Immunogenicity

Two areas of continuing concern are anti-drug antibody and long-term pharmacovigilance. Unlike the EU requirements, no specific post-marketing pharmacovigilance plan is required in the US ODAC advisors felt that routine pharmacovigilance, supported by unique product names, and the absence of interchangeability would facilitate pharmacovigilance, particularly in cancer and HIV settings.

2.1.16 Lessons from the European Union (EU) Countries

In the EU, regulatory approval was granted for five biosimilar epoetins between 2007 and 2008. Epoetin biosimilars differ in degree of glycosylation, which affects pharmacokinetics, pharmacodynamics, effectiveness, safety, and immunogenicity. Approvals were based on the totality of evidence concepts, as in the United States. Multi-dose and single-dose biosimilar epoetin vials are approved (versus single-dose vials only in the United States). Biosimilar epoetins all have the same mechanisms of action, although pharmacological properties differ. Most approvals were based on the demonstration of comparability with the Eprex formulation, a formulation marketed outside the United States. For three biosimilar epoetins, extrapolations were granted for all indications approved for reference epoetin in the United States and the EU. Two biosimilars have three indications—the same as the reference epoetin evaluated by regulatory agencies.

Differences in biosimilar epoetins usage vary by country, primarily related to regional differences in payment systems. In 2011, the use of biosimilar epoetins was greater than first- and second-generation reference epoetins in Sweden and Germany, but uptake in Italy, France, and the United Kingdom was not. Price discounting is limited in some countries. Some hypothesize that the slow uptake of biosimilars reflects efficacy and safety concerns. However, no unexpected side effects are identified with the EU biosimilar epoetins.

The biosimilar epoetin EU country discounts range from 20 to 35%. Greece, Finland, and Germany are the largest users of biosimilar epoetins with adoption earlier than the other EU countries. German insurance funds have biosimilar epoetin prescribing targets because pricing for reference biologicals is high. German physicians view biosimilar epoetins favorably. Physicians in other EU countries are less supportive. In some countries—e.g., Finland and France—hospitals adopted financial incentives for biosimilar epoetins because hospitals pay for in-hospital but not outpatient drugs. Germany established reference pricing and specific regional quotas for physicians and sickness funds for biosimilar epoetins. Spain has not adopted biosimilar epoetins because prescribing decisions are made regionally by local physicians.

2.1.17 Lessons from Japan

In 2010, Japan granted regulatory authority for biosimilar epoetin for use for renal anemia and anemia of prematurity. Japan did not grant regulatory approval for use in cancer chemotherapy anemia as the reference epoetin (ESPO ®) does not have regulatory approval for this indication. Epoetin biosimilar in Japan (epoetin alfa BS [JCR]) was originally developed as a new molecular entity. During product development, Japanese guidelines for follow-on biologics were published and the licensure strategy was changed to a follow-on biologic. The clinical data package of Epoetin alfa BS [JCR] included a Phase I study assessing the PK profile in healthy volunteers. Two cross-over studies comparing safety and PK profile of epoetin alfa BS [JCR] and reference epoetin (ESPO®) were conducted using intravenous and subcutaneous administration. A Phase II/III study was a randomized, double-blind, parallel-group, multicenter design study in 329 hemodialysis patients with renal anemia comparing efficacy and safety between epoetin alfa BS [JCR] and reference epoetin. A long-term single-arm study confirmed the long-term safety and efficacy of epoetin alfa BS [JCR] in 143 hemodialysis patients with renal anemia. There was no significant difference between epoetin alfa BS [JCR] and ESPO® regarding efficacy, adverse events, and serious adverse events. No instances of anti-EPO antibody development were identified. Clinical studies of epeotin alfa BS [JCR] evaluated patients on hemodialysis in a maintenance phase. Clinical data about patients on peritoneal dialysis and in a correction phase were not collected and clinical studies of anemia for premature infants were not conducted (although reference product ESPO® has two indications—renal anemia undergoing dialysis and anemia of prematurity). It was possible to extrapolate from renal anemia undergoing hemodialysis to the two indications of the reference epoetin since the mechanism of action is the same.

2.2 Conclusions

The first US biosimilar epoetin received an ODAC recommendation for FDA licensing approval in May 2017. The decision for FDA approval occurred in 2018. The 2017 application was an amended submission of an application that was reportedly not approved in part because a manufacturing process resulted in a greater amount of EPO in each vial compared to reference epoetin. After altering its manufacturing processes, the current submission corrected this problem. The sponsor, FDA reviewers, and ODAC identified some areas in the submission where residual uncertainty remained, such as differences in glycosylation. Later studies identified no clinical relevance for these differences. As with all approved biosimilars in the United States, before marketing occurs, patent litigation was completed. This case determined that biosimilar epoetin marketing could begin in 2018. After that, favorable pricing to dialysis centers and oncology practices encouraged usage as well as favorable formulary placements by large insurers. Overall, price discounts were not transparent, but appear to be in the range of 20%– 30%. At this time, other biosimilar epoteins are not expected to apply for FDA approval with the advent of new types of anemia-treating agents. However, the success in licensing and litigation challenges and marketing enhanced competition, lowered prices, and achieved high market penetration for biosimilar epoetin. In the United States, competition is the principal factor that determines if biosimilar epoetin may bend the healthcare cost curve back. Long-term experiences from the EU and Japan, where national health insurance programs negotiate substantial discounts, and emerging experiences from the United States suggest that high market penetration may facilitate biosimilar epoetin in bending the cancer cost curve. Initial pessimism that biosimilars will bend the cost curve appears to be dissipating.

References

1. Kozlowski S, Woodcock J, Midthun K, Sherman RB (2011) Developing the nation's biosimilars program. N Engl J Med 365:385–388
2. Bennett CL, Chen B, Hermanson T et al (2014) Regulatory and clinical considerations for biosimilar oncology drugs. Lancet Oncol 15(13):e594–e605
3. Schellekens H, Smolen JS, Dicato M, Rifkin RM (2016) Safety and efficacy of biosimilars in oncology. Lancet Oncol 17:e502–e509
4. IMS Institute for Helathcare Informatics (2014) Assessing biologic uptake and competition in European markets. http://www.imhealth.com/files/web/IMS%20InstituteHealtcare%20Briefs/Assessing_Biosimilar_uptake_and_competition_in_Europeanmarkets.pdf. Accessed 20 Dec 2016
5. Food and Drug Administration (2016) Labeling for biosimilar products: guidance for industry. http://www.fda.gov/downloads/drugs/guidancecomplianceregulatoryinformation/guidances/ucm493439.pdf. Accessed 8 April 2017
6. Sato D (2016) Surging the wave in Japan for regulatory convergence of biosimilar. http://www.egaevents.org/presentations/2016bios/Daisaku_Sato.pdf. Accessed 15 Dec 2016
7. National Conference of State Legislatures (2017) State laws and regulations related to biologic medications and substitutions of biosimilars. http://www.ncsl.org/research/health/state-laws-and-legislation-related-to-biologic-medications-and-substitution-of-biosimilars.aspx. Accessed 17 April 2017
8. Arato T (2016) Japanese regulation of biosimilar products: past experience and current challenges. Br J Clin Pharmacol 82:130–140

Sumimasa Nagai MD Ph.D. is deputy director of the Translational Research Center of the University of Tokyo Hospital and clinical expert advisor at Companion Diagnostics Working Group and the Office of New Drugs V (oncology) at the Pharmaceuticals and Medical Devices Agency in Japan. At PMDA, he has been involved in regulating oncologic drugs and companion diagnostics. He has been a lead author on Lancet Oncology pieces on oncology biosimilar medications and on additional articles on biosimilar epoetin and filgrastim in collaboration with Dr. Bennett and the SONAR group.

Bartlett J. Witherspoon MBA is a third-year medical student at the Medical University of South Carolina and a graduate of Vanderbilt University's Master's in Business Administration program. He is an active co-investigator with Dr. Bennett and the SONAR project and has been a lead co-investigator on published manuscripts on fluoroquinolone-associated disability and on biosimilar oncology products.

Dr. Chadi Nabhan is a Hematologist and Medical Oncologist with special interests in malignant hematology as well as GU malignancies. He did two years of basic science research at Massachusetts General Hospital/Harvard Medical School before completing his residency at Loyola University in Chicago and a fellowship at Northwestern University and Robert H. Lurie Comprehensive Cancer Center. He holds an MBA in Health Care Management from Loyola University Quinlan School of Business.

Charles L. Bennett MD Ph.D. MPPSmartState Chair and Frank P. and Josie M. Fletcher Chair of Medication Safety and Efficacy and Director, SmartState Center for Medication Safety and Efficacy, is also a Visiting Scholar at the City of Hope National Cancer Institute Designated Comprehensive Cancer Center in Duarte, California and is the co-editor of this book, Cancer Policy (2nd Edition). Dr. Bennett is a Phi Beta Kappa and High Honors graduate in mathematics from Swarthmore College, earned his medical degree in 1981 from the University of Pennsylvania

Perelman School of Medicine, and completed internal medicine, hematology, and oncology training at the Michael Reese Hospital and the University of Chicago Pritzger School of Medicine before completing his PhD and Masters In Public Policy degrees with honors in social science at the RAND Pardee Graduate School of Public Policy in Santa Monica, California. He has led a 20-year National Institutes of Health funded pharmacovigilance called the Research on Adverse Drug events And Reports (RADAR) and subsequently called to Southern Network on Adverse drug Reactions (SONAR) at the University of South Carolina College of Pharmacy.

Policing of Drug Safety Information Dissemination Under the False Claims Act

Brian Chen, Tony Yang, and Charles L. Bennett

3.1 Introduction

On July 25, 2017, the second largest multi-million dollar settlement was pursued with the assistance of the Department of Justice and alleging inappropriate marketing strategies utilized by the pharmaceutical industry came to an end [1]. Federal prosecutors announced that the pharmaceutical manufacturing company, Celgene Corporation, would pay $280 million to resolve allegations surrounding: off-label promotion of thalidomide and lenalidomide, its first two billion dollar cancer drugs; failure to adequately disseminate pharmaceutical safety information via its pharmaceutical representatives; and facilitation of ghost writing efforts by PhD consultants for key opinion leaders [1]. Beverly Brown who had been a sales representative until 2007 had filed the case, *United States ex rel. Brown v. Celgene*, in California in 2007. This case was dismissed with summary judgement, only to be reinstated by Ms. Brown with support of a team of three law firms (from Washington DC, Los Angeles, and Columbia, South Carolina) in 2010 [1]. Ms. Brown alleged that the manufacturer had violated the Federal False Claims Act ("FCA") as well numerous analogous state False Claims Acts (related to Medicaid sales of pharmaceuticals) by heavily marketing thalidomide and lenalidomide for numerous cancers for which the immune-modulatory drugs had not received FDA approval to treat and furthermore that the manufacturer had offered numerous financial incentives to key opinion leaders who in turn would promote expanded use of the two

B. Chen · T. Yang · C. L. Bennett (✉)
SONAR (Southern Network on Adverse Reactions) Program, University of South Carolina College of Pharmacy, Columbia, SC 29208, USA
e-mail: bennettc@cop.sc.edu

B. Chen
e-mail: bchen@mailbox.sc.edu

T. Yang
e-mail: ytyyang@email.gwu.edu

drugs [1]. Most of the settlement was paid to the federal government while 28 states and the District of Columbia received $20.7 million [1]. The magnitude of this financial settlement, coupled with the failure to assign criminal liability to any employee of the company, strongly suggests a need for regulatory reform [1].

3.1.1 The Settlement

In April 2010, a former "immunology specialist" for Celgene (Beverly Brown) brought a $40 billion FCA lawsuit against Celgene Corporation in the United States District Court for the Central District of California. Celgene had hired "immunology specialists" as their main pharmaceutical product sales representatives at that time as thalidomide, was an immunological treatment for cutaneous manifestations of leprosy and the company did not have FDA approval for thalidomide or lenalidomide as a cancer therapy. Three years previously, she had become concerned when her manager had reportedly advised Ms. Brown to change billing codes on physician's insurance claims to reflect diagnoses for which thalidomide and lenalidomide had been approved (multiple myeloma for thalidomide after May 2006 and leprosy prior to that time and myelodysplastic syndrome for lenalidomide after May 2005 and multiple myeloma after May 2006) and to remove billing codes for other cancer diagnoses. These allegations claimed that the manufacturer had developed a large program for promoting thalidomide and lenalidomide for a wide range of cancer diagnoses for which the drugs had not been approved at the time of the promotion effort [2]. In particularly, Ms. Brown asserted that her manager as well as other managers of the company had advised that the "immunology specialists" promote the use of the two drugs to treat numerous cancers, including breast cancer, prostate cancer, and chronic lymphocytic leukemia, and that after physicians had filed claims that included altered insurance codes, federal and state government programs ultimately paid for such off-label uses. In her deposition for the case, Ms. Brown alleged that Celgene offered financial inducements to key physician opinion leaders who had support this marketing strategy, paying physicians speaker fees as much as $6,000 for a single day of consulting and had also made $50 million to $100 million donations annually to patient assistance funds called to the Patient Access Network and the Chronic Disease Fund to allow patients to forego copayment requirements (the mean annual cost of thalidomide was in the range of $10,000 annually) [3]. According to Ms. Brown, these initiatives had transformed Celgene from a small business with virtually no pharmaceutical products to a pharmaceutical giant that was recently purchased by Bristol Myers Squibb for $76 billion [3]. Allegations of payments to the patient assistance funds were not included in the actual lawsuit filed by Brown and her qui tam attorneys, however.

When the facts of the case were first unsealed in 2014 following an extensive investigation by the qui tam lawyers (the United States federal Department of Justice attorneys had declined to intervene), attorneys for Celgene from Jones Day moved for summary judgment and refuted each of Brown's claims [3]. Specifically, the attorneys argued that Federal government Medicare officials had known that off-label uses of thalidomide and lenalidomide in the oncology setting represented the then majority of the use of these drugs as their initial FDA marketing approvals in 1998 (for leprosy) and 2005 (for myelodysplastic syndrome), but had continued to provide reimbursement when the drugs were purchased by insurance programs, including Medicare and Medicaid [4]. The Jones Day attorneys cited the United States' Supreme Court's decision in *Universal Health Services, Inc. v. United States ex rel. Escobar*, stating that the government's decisions to reimburse for off-label uses of thalidomide and lenalidomide were made with full knowledge that these uses were off-label [4]. The attorneys characterized off-label promotion of thalidomide and lenalidomide as being protected by free speech considerations under the First Amendment. They cited several court decisions that purportedly supported supporting this position. In response, the qui tam attorneys for Ms. Brown opined that the Second Circuit's ruling in *United States v. Caronia* was not controlling law in California, the state where the federal case had been filed, and that therefore the manufacturer had forfeited its constitutional safeguards by misleadingly concealing from providers the severe safety risks of venous thromboembolism that had been identified by the Research on Adverse Drug Events and Reports (RADAR) project from Northwestern University (led by Charles L Bennett MD PhD MPP) [3].

The litigation proved a massive undertaking, encompassing more than 40 depositions, 12,000 pages of transcripts, and over six million documents [3]. At the close of the discovery period on December 28, 2016, District Court Judge George King issued an order denying summary judgement in part, dismissing the kickback claims as well as allegations related to claims submitted to the Veterans Administration, the U.S. Defense Health Agency, and the Medicaid programs of Tennessee, Texas, and Wisconsin [3]. Although the government had declined to intervene in the case, the Department of Justice ("DOJ") filed a statement of interest. Accusing the company of misrepresenting Medicaid reimbursement standards and the burden of proof for FCA relators, the government was largely critical of Celgene's marketing practices and legal position [4].

On July 17, 2017, the three attorney groups for Ms. Brown and Jones Day attorneys who represented Celgene filed under seal a joint motion for settlement approval [4]. Jones Day attorneys continued to allege that Celgene denied any wrongdoing in the case, affirming that the usual statement one notes with any settlement (the company settled to avoid the uncertainty, distractions, and expense of protracted litigation) applied here [4]. The formal settlement text suggests otherwise, as it includes detailed statements alleging that Celgene promoted thalidomide and lenalidomide for uses that were both unapproved and unsafe and had also offered kickbacks to influence key physician opinion leaders and other physicians to prescribe these two drugs regardless of reimbursement potential or medical necessity [4]. The final resolution included allegations that Celgene had purposefully concealed adverse events associated with the medications, such as venous thromboembolism, and, through payments to key physician opinion leaders, the published drug compendia, medical literature, and published clinical studies supported unproven uses that (at the time of the filing of the lawsuit) for these two drugs [4].

3.1.2 Lessons Learned and Legal Precedent

The settlement of this qui tam litigation provides further support that when several hundred million-dollar settlements are agreed upon by a multi-billion-dollar pharmaceutical company such as Celgene, a criminal finding against specific corporate executives should be considered. These findings are particularly important in civil qui tam lawsuits that involved allegations of significant safety risks that were experienced by large numbers of patients. There has been a transition in the qui tam lawsuit cases away from allegations of off-label marketing to allegations of failing to adequately inform patients and physicians of safety concerns of pharmaceuticals —as exemplified by the multitude of federal and state cases involving opioids. Recently, federal authorities charged Laurence Doud III, the Chief Executive Officer of Rochester Drug Cooperative of conspiracy to traffic narcotics and defrauding the federal government by not reporting suspicious pharmaceutical activities to the Drug Enforcement Agency. It should be noted that the large number of high-dollar and high-profile qui tam settlements, including several that allege failure to adequately report drug safety concerns, argues strongly that a primary deterrent to protect patient safety would be to criminally charge one or more pharmaceutical executives in these cases [4].

Attorneys who focus on off-label marketing, rather than drug safety, allege that statutes and regulations that guide pharmaceutical and medical device promotion are unconstitutional [4]. They argue that the First Amendment does not limit free flow of scientific information, including information about off-label drug usage, even if this information supports medical uses that are not approved by the FDA and which, in fact, may be neither safe nor effective [4] In *Sorrell v. IMS Health*, the United States' Supreme Court ruled as unconstitutional state laws that bar pharmaceutical companies from accessing data of physician prescribing patterns for marketing purposes [4]. In the 2012 case of *United States v. Caronia*, the Second Circuit ruled that a criminal conviction of a sales representative for misbranding based upon truthful off-label promotion violated the Constitution [4]. In 2015, Amarin Pharma brought a First Amendment challenge against the ban regarding off-label promotion of pharmaceuticals. The attorneys for Amarin argued that the company had a constitutional right to promote its omega-3 fatty acid based on off-label, but truthful, claim that inconclusive research had demonstrated that consumption may reduce the risk of coronary heart disease [4]. The FDA's 2015 response was the FDA was not concerned about most of the material that the company had proposed to communicate and therefore did not consider the dissemination of this material false or misleading [4]. The District Court, ruling in favor of Amarin, issued preliminary relief and allowed the manufacturer to promote material that was deemed as truthful and non-misleading [4]. The actual implications of these decisions have been viewed as narrow, and unlikely to inform broad policy decisions [4].

A major lesson learned from the Celgene case is that the current regulatory regime is both under-enforced and ineffective. Due to ever increasing pharmaceutical prices, an increasing number of drugs for which safety concerns have been overlooked for decades, and the high rate of overprescribing and misprescribing of pharmaceuticals, pharmaceutical companies are increasingly viewed as being able to include multi-billion dollar settlements with the government as a "cost of doing business" [2]. For instance, when Celgene paid $280 million to settle the FCA violations civil allegations, this amount was viewed by many as a necessary cost of doing business as the company moved toward its $76 billion purchase by Bristol Myers Squibb. In response to a Citizen Petition jointly filed in 2005 by Charles L Bennett MD PhD MPP and then Connecticut Attorney General Richard Blumenthal (now a Connecticut senator), attorneys for Celgene negotiated in 2006 with the FDA promises that the company would actively educate clinicians about venous thromboembolism associated with thalidomide and lenalidomide—safety concerns that were included extensively in the 2017 settlement between US Attorneys and Beverly Brown with Celgene.

3.1.3 Future of Policing Drug Safety Efforts

Some have suggested that targeting individual executives within offending drug companies could prove a more effective method of enforcing the FCA and FDA's requirements that pharmaceutical manufacturers must effectively provide accurate information on pharmaceutical safety [2]. In criminally prosecuting or excluding executives from participation in federal insurance programs including Medicare, policymakers posit that patient safety might increase and real patient benefits might occur [2]. In 2011, the former chief executive of K.V. Pharmaceutical received 30 days in jail and a $1 million fine for selling unsafe and misbranded morphine tablets that included more milligrams of the active pharmaceutical ingredients than was printed on the drug label—thus opening patients up to acute overdosing, respiratory depression, coma, and death [2]. A similar approach to FCA cases might encourage management to more actively police under- and misleading promotion of pharmaceutical safety concerns within their companies [2].

More practicable reform proposals emphasize the need for increased transparency in disseminating safety information to providers and patients [2]. Many prescriptions paid for by Medicare Part D and state Medicaid programs are not accompanied by information regarding the patient's diagnosis, thus making it difficult if not impossible to address safety concerns that might occur in specific disease states, such as progressive multifocal leukoencephalopathy with rituximab-treatment of non-Hodgkin's lymphoma [2]. To reduce the number of claims that are filed where safety concerns are not readily apparent, lawmakers and regulators might consider requiring pharmacists to provide this information just as physicians do when submitting claims to Medicare Part B [2]. This would eliminate the lengthy process necessary to uncover serious adverse drug reactions that occur when pharmaceuticals are administered in some settings but not in other clinical settings, requiring the government to match a patient's treatment history to a claim for reimbursement and to show that the patient's diagnosis is not a medically accepted indication for the prescribed drug [2]. What is more, such reform would enhance the ability of federal and state regulators to improve drug safety and decrease the extent of false claims that are associated with misbranded drugs that include incorrect or insufficient safety language [2].

In further delineating the contours of its focus on pharmaceutical safety, the FDA would clarify manufacturer exposure to direct enforcement and liability resulting from "misbranding" [2]. By "passing legislation, promulgating regulations, issuing guidance documents, developing safe harbors, or implementing an advisory opinion process," FDA should provide clear standards to companies attempting to disseminate accurate information about the safety of their pharmaceuticals [2]. Increased enforcement by the FDA might also lead to more immediate corrections of problematic safety-focused activities and better results leveraging FDA's expertise in the area of pharmaceutical safety [2].

Finally, by enhancing transparency of enforcement and settlement terms, interested parties could easily ascertain whether there has been wrongdoing by a company, whether a case has been treated criminally or civilly, and how much financial penalty and/or criminal jail sentences should be evaluated if there has been wrongdoing [2]. This would encourage qui tam relators to bring lawsuits related to pharmaceutical safety concerns while providing the industry more explicit rules related to drug safety information dissemination to which they must conform [2]. In providing information about the government's reasoning in negotiating and arriving at settlement amounts and rationale for filing criminal charges, regulators and the Department of Justice could dispel the notion that such penalties are "the costs of doing business" [2]. Through the implementation of these and other similar reforms, the government could reduce the number of false claims cases that focus on misbranding and drug safety concerns.

3.2 Conclusion

The recent multi-million-dollar settlement between Celgene and the federal government aptly illustrates the growing problem of pharmaceutical safety and poor information dissemination efforts by pharmaceutical manufacturers [2]. Reform efforts calling for increased transparency in establishing rules for and pursuing violations of the FCA related to misinformation of pharmaceutical safety concerns have the potential to promote patient safety [2]. Both Congress and the FDA must take steps to ensure that such measures are put in place in the immediate future to reduce fraud and wasted taxpayer resources and to prevent loss of patient lives.

References

1. PR Newswire (2017) Bio pharma giant—celgene—settles case alleging marketing violations for $280 million, Markets Insider (July 25, 2017). http://markets.businessinsider.com/news/stocks/Bio-Pharma-Giant-Celgene-Settles-Case-Alleging-Marketing-Violations-For-280-Million-1002203763
2. Melissa Daniels, Celgene to Pay $280 Million to End Off-Label Cancer Drug FCA Suit, Law360 (July 25, 2017). https://www-law360-com.mutex.gmu.edu/articles/948014?scroll=1
3. Department of Justice, Celgene agrees to pay $280 Million to resolve fraud allegations, (July 24, 2017). https://www.justice.gov/usao-cdca/pr/celgene-agrees-pay-280-million-resolve-fraud-allegations-related-promotion-cancer-drugs (Accessed Oct 18, 2022).
4. Reuters, Celgene agrees to settle $280 million off-label marketing. litigation, (July 27, 2017). https://www.reuters.com/article/us-celgene-lawsuit-idUKKBN1AA2PA (Accessed Oct 18, 2022).

Brian Chen JD Ph.D. is an Associate Professor with tenure at the Arnold School of Public Health at the University of South Carolina and a leading policy investigator on cancer-related safety concerns. His education is from Harvard College, Stanford School of Law, and the University of California, Berkeley Ph.D. program in economics under Paul Gertler Ph.D., Professor, the University of California. Dr. Chen has led several initiatives to file Citizen Petitions with the FDA, and he has been an active, funded R01 co-investigator on the SONAR project.

Tony Yang ScD LLM MPH, Professor, George Washington School of Nursing in Washington DC is trained in health services research and law at Harvard University. He is executive director for Center for Health Policy and Media Engagement at the George Washington University School of Nursing and holds a joint appointment in the Department of Health Policy and Management. He received the Early Career Award for Excellence in Public Health Law from the American Public Health Association. He holds graduate degrees in public health from the TS Chan School of Public Health at Harvard University, health policy at the School of Public Policy at Harvard University, and law from the University of Pennsylvania. He has led several SONAR projects on health care law and pharmaceuticals.

Charles L. Bennett MD Ph.D. MPP, SmartState Chair and Frank P and Josie M Fletcher Chair of Medication Safety and Efficacy and Director, SmartState Center for Medication Safety and Efficacy, is also a Visiting Scholar at the City of Hope National Cancer Institute Designated Comprehensive Cancer Center in Duarte, California and is the co-editor of this book, Cancer Policy (2nd Edition). Dr. Bennett is a Phi Beta Kappa and High Honors graduate in mathematics from Swarthmore College, earned his medical degree in 1981 from the University of Pennsylvania Perelman School of Medicine, and completed internal medicine, hematology, and oncology training at the Michael Reese Hospital and the University of Chicago Pritzger School of Medicine before completing his Ph.D. and Masters In Public Policy degrees with honors in social science at the RAND Pardee Graduate School of Public Policy in Santa Monica, California. He has led a 20-year National Institutes of Health funded pharmacovigilance called the Research on Adverse Drug events And Reports (RADAR) and subsequently called to Southern Network on Adverse drug Reactions (SONAR) at the University of South Carolina College of Pharmacy.

Translating Research into Health Policy: The Citizen Petition Experience with the Food and Drug Administration

4

Paul Ray and Charles L. Bennett

4.1 Introduction

Translating research findings into policy is important. Health policy researchers often testify before Congressional subcommittees and provide background on health policy issues. A rarely used, but important, tool for facilitating the translation of research into policy is via filing a Citizen Petition. Based on the First Amendment right of citizens to "petition the Government for a redress of grievances," Title 21, section 10.30 of the Code of Federal Regulations stipulates that citizens may request the Food and Drug Administration (FDA) to "issue, amend, or revoke a regulation or order or take or refrain from taking any other form of administrative action" [1]. Citizen Petitions filed with the FDA have the potential to protect the public's health if the Petitions lead to improved pharmaceutical safety. A Citizen Petition must include a description of actions being requested, and these actions must fall under the jurisdiction of the FDA commissioner. Each petition must include persuasive statements of grounds such as data from randomized, controlled trials, a statement on environmental and economic impacts (if any), and certification that the evidence included is well balanced and unbiased.

Between 2001 and 2013, 1915 Citizen Petitions were filed with the FDA [2, 3]. Of these, 82% were filed by individuals working for industry. Most petitions focused on blocking or delaying FDA approval of generic products [4]. In contrast, 130 citizen petitions were filed by individuals or organizations not working on behalf of the pharmaceutical industry. These Citizen Petitions usually requested labeling changes, addition or removal of boxed warnings, risk communications, or

P. Ray · C. L. Bennett (✉)
SONAR (Southern Network on Adverse Reactions) Program, University of South Carolina College of Pharmacy, Columbia, SC 29208, USA
e-mail: bennettc@cop.sc.edu

P. Ray
e-mail: bossdoc2@comcast.net

C. Bennett et al. (eds.), *Cancer Drug Safety and Public Health Policy*,
Cancer Treatment and Research 184, https://doi.org/10.1007/978-3-031-04402-1_4

placement of drugs into a Risk Evaluation and Mitigation Strategy. Twenty-three Citizen Petitions filed with the FDA by non-profit organizations or individuals resulted in safety actions such as addition of Boxed warnings, withdrawal of marketing approval of unsafe drugs, or a pharmaceutical manufacturer initiating a Risk Evaluation and Management Strategy (REMS). Of 23 successful Citizen Petitions, 19 were filed by public advocacy programs such as Public Citizen, medical specialty groups, or paid consultants to pharmaceutical manufacturers [2, 3]. Four successful Citizen Petitions were filed by health policy researchers. Herein, we review these four Citizen Petitions, the stated rationale for filing these Citizen Petitions, substance of the FDA Response Letters, and actions taken by the FDA and manufacturers. Finally, recommendations to improve the Citizen Petition process are outlined.

As summarized previously, we reviewed 1,915 citizen petitions filed with the FDA from 2001 to 2013 [2, 3]. These petitions are publicly available at www. regulations.gov, and searchable using the term "FDA-YEAR-P." Petitions with a final FDA decision include a Response Letter in which a senior employee of the FDA details the nature of the petition requests, the reasoning for the decision, and in instances where partial or full approval has been decided, a detailed independent review of data that address the response. In total, 130 FDA Citizen Petitions were filed by individuals or organizations other than manufacturers. Four Citizen Petitions were filed by researchers and received partial or full approval and several FDA actions were undertaken for each of these Petitions.

Information on submission/decision dates, outcome, petitioners, and reasons for decisions was extracted from the FDA decision letters available in the docket folder for each approved citizen petition (available at regulations.gov). Information on actions taken by the pharmaceutical manufacturer and the FDA was abstracted. For the pharmaceutical manufacturer, data were abstracted on the following activities if performed in response to the Citizen Petition: issuance of a Dear Doctor or Dear Doctor letter, specific edits of sections and text of product label revisions (available at drugs@FDA for each drug), the initiation and outcome of any Post-marketing Commitment studies, and issuance or edits of Medication Guides. For manufacturers of pharmaceuticals in the same therapeutic class as the drug that was the focus of the Citizen Petition, similar data were abstracted. For the FDA, data were abstracted on independent data analyses conducted by FDA related to the Citizen Petition, FDA analytic review of data included in Citizen Petition, Public Health Advisories, Drug Safety Communications, and tasks assigned to the manufacturer related to the specific drug identified in the Citizen Petition as well as for other drugs in the same therapeutic class. Additional data on FDA responses and rationale for Citizen Petitions were abstracted from published case study descriptions for the thalidomide and metformin Citizen Petitions [2, 5].

4.1.1 The Citizen Petitions

The first successful Citizen Petition, from a hematologist and health policy research scientist Charles Bennett, was filed in 2005 in collaboration with then Connecticut Attorney General Richard Blumenthal [3]. The Petition requested that FDA require the manufacturer of thalidomide revise the product label to indicate that up to 25% of cancer patients who received thalidomide for multiple myeloma had developed life-threatening venous thromboembolism [6]. The Petition also requested that physicians consider prescribing aspirin or an anti-thrombotic agent in conjunction with thalidomide and corticosteroids. National Institute of Health funded research had identified the adverse event that was the focus of the Petition. In 2006, Blumenthal received a response letter from Steve Galson MD MPH, then Director of FDA's Center for Drug Evaluation and Research [7]. Dr. Galson indicated that the FDA agreed in part with the Citizen Petition. In May 2006, the manufacturer revised its product label along the lines requested in the Petition. Factual evidence supporting the Petition was a meta-analysis prepared by the hematologist that identified a 30% increased venous thromboembolism risk when thalidomide was administered to persons with a wide range of cancers [1]. FDA's response, based on an independent meta-analysis of thalidomide administration to persons with multiple myeloma, identified a 25% increased venous thromboembolism risk.

The second successful Citizen Petition from a health policy research scientist was filed in 2009 by Dennis Cotter, the President of a non-profit organization (Medical Technologies and Practice Patterns Institute).[MTPPI] Citizen Petition 2009] The organization monitored patterns of use of erythropoiesis stimulating agents (ESAs) by two manufacturers who competitively marketed ESAs. Cotter requested that the FDA require the manufacturer of the erythropoiesis stimulating agent (ESA) to revise Black Box warnings indicating that administration of high ESA doses to chronic kidney disease patients would lead to increased risks of death and myocardial infarction and that ESA administration targeting high serum hemoglobin levels was associated with the same risks. In 2011, Janet Woodcock MD, the Director of the FDA's Center for Drug Evaluation and Research FDA, informed Cotter that the FDA had required ESA manufacturers to revise ESA Boxed Warnings to indicate that no clinical trial had identified a target hemoglobin level, ESA dose, or ESA dosing strategy that was not associated with increased risks of death, myocardial infarctions, or stroke [8]. The factual evidence supporting the Citizen Petition included a review of three randomized clinical trials with ESAs that identified toxicity risks and additional database analyses identifying risks of death, myocardial infarction, and stroke among ESA-treated persons with end stage renal disease. FDA's response indicated that they independently identified the same safety concerns based on their review of the same three clinical trial reports described in the Citizen Petition and one clinical trial report published after the Citizen Petition had been filed.

The third and fourth successful Citizen Petitions from research scientists were filed by academic clinicians and researchers at medical universities at Cornell University, Yale University, and the University of Pennsylvania [5, 9, 10]. The

Citizen Petitions, while similar in content, were filed months apart in 2012 and 2013. The Citizen Petition from the Yale clinicians requested that the product label be revised to remove a Box warning describing lactic acidosis occurring with metformin. The Citizen Petition from clinicians and researchers at the University of Pennsylvania and Cornell Weill requested that the contra-indication section of the metformin label be revised to indicate that metformin should be considered in persons with creatinine clearance >60 ml per minute per 1.73 square meters. Janet Woodcock, the Director of the Center for Drug Evaluation of Research at FDA responded in 2016 to both Petitions in a single letter indicating that FDA denied the Yale request to revise the Black Box label, while accepting other Yale requests for revisions in other sections of the product label [11]. The FDA noted that the Penn/Cornell Petition recommended changes in the contra-indication section of the label to indicate that metformin was contra-indicated only among metformin-treated persons with severe renal insufficiency. The existing FDA label indicated that metformin was contra-indicated in patients with mild, moderate, or severe renal insufficiency. Dr. Woodcock's letter indicated that the FDA reviewed background information cited in both Petitions and additional literature on metformin and lactic acidosis.

4.2 Conclusions

Having gone through four Citizen Petitions from research scientists that were granted in part by the FDA and for which FDA and manufacturers implemented safety-related responses, what lessons have been learned and what are the future implications?

First, preparing a competitive Citizen Petition required a significant investment of time, personnel, funds, and persons with close relationships with FDA or Congress. Successful Petitions were based on NIH-funded R01 research (two petitions) or a NIH training grant (for metformin) that provided the evidence basis for the requests. Unpublished draft research papers were included in the submissions. For these Petitions, a year after the Petition was filed, data included in the Citizen Petitions were published in medical journals. Recommendations to file these Petitions came from then Connecticut Attorney General Blumenthal (thalidomide), a senior economist at the Center for Medicare and Medicaid Services (ESAs), a director of FDA's Division for Endocrinology Products (the metformin Petition from clinicians in the Departments of Medicine at Yale University and Cornell University), and the Deputy Director of the FDA's Center for Drug Evaluation and Research (the Penn petition on metformin) [5]. Teams of persons who developed these grants included clinicians, policy analysts, and statisticians. For ESAs, a senior Center for Medicare and Medicaid services economist developed an economic impact statement (identifying a potential $8 billion annual saving). For thalidomide, Connecticut Attorney General Blumenthal raised concerns that FDA-approved product labels did not provide warnings for side effects that occur in "off-label" clinical settings and as such, a state Attorney General had a public health obligation to fill that void. For the metformin Petition filed by clinicians and researchers from the University of Pennsylvania, support letters from nine endocrinologists accompanied the Petition and identified a long-standing clinical concern that metformin was safe to use in settings that the existing product label had identified as unsafe [12].

Second, evidentiary material submitted with each Citizen Petition required months to prepare. For thalidomide, a literature-based meta-analysis was included in the Citizen Petition. For ESAs, a data base analysis of mortality among Medicare covered persons with chronic kidney disease on dialysis who received versus did not receive epoetin was submitted to the FDA. For the metformin submission from clinicians and researchers at Cornell Weill Medical School, results of a phase III clinical trial identifying safety with metformin administration to persons with mild renal insufficiency were submitted. For the metformin Citizen Petition from clinicians and researchers at Yale and the University of Pennsylvania Medical Schools, a analysis identifying better characterization of renal insufficiency with estimated Glomerular Filtration Rate (eGFR) measurement than serum creatinine was included.

Third, FDA responses required months to years to prepare. The one-year response time for the thalidomide response was the shortest response time and was facilitated by simultaneous FDA review of the manufacturer's dossier seeking regulatory approval for treatment of multiple myeloma, representing a new clinical indication for thalidomide. FDA reviewers in the Division of Drug Marketing and Communication were independently evaluating the manufacturer's proposed product label statements on venous thromboembolism. FDA statisticians in the Office of Safety and Epidemiology were completing a meta-analysis of venous thromboembolism rates in phase III clinical trials for multiple myeloma patients who received thalidomide and corticosteroids. The unexpected simultaneous submission of Blumenthal's Citizen Petition and the manufacturer's request for marketing approval for thalidomide resulted in a large number of FDA personnel reviewing safety considerations, although independently. In 2006, when FDA reviewers decided to grant marketing approval for thalidomide as a treatment of multiple myeloma, personnel with the Division of Drug Marketing and Communication reported that thalidomide-associated venous thromboembolism was incompletely addressed in the proposed product label. After a revised product label was submitted by the manufacturer and reviewed and approved by FDA's Director of the Center for Drug Research and Evaluation, marketing approval and a partial approval for the Citizen Petition were simultaneously announced in May 2006.

Fourth, follow-up activities from the FDA and the relevant manufacturers were extensive and timely [13, 14]. FDA communicated directly with manufacturers, informing the manufacturers of required changes in the product label. Manufacturers then revised Boxed Warnings, warnings, and indications sections of various product labels, and disseminated Dear Healthcare Provider letters and revised Medication Guides. (By regulation, pharmaceutical manufacturers are required to respond to FDA requests for changes in product labels, issuance of Dear Healthcare

Providers, and design of requested Post-Marketing Commitment studies within 30 days). FDA disseminated Drug Safety Communications to providers within months of sending Response Letters to the Petitioners outlining required product label changes. FDA communicated their concerns to manufacturers of all pharmaceuticals in the same class for thalidomide (lenalidomide) and for epoetin (darbepoetin). For erythropoiesis stimulating agents, FDA also hosted a Podcast for Healthcare Professionals in 2011[FDA ESA Podcase].

Fifth, research included in the Citizen Petitions was subsequently published in the literature. The thalidomide Citizen Petition was followed three months later by a JAMA publication of the meta-analysis [1]. The meta-analysis in the Citizen Petition described thalidomide-associated venous thromboembolism in the oncology setting, while the JAMA publication described thalidomide- and lenalidomide-associated venous thromboembolism in the setting of multiple myeloma. The 2009 ESA Citizen Petition was based on some of the Petitioner's large database study published in JAMA in 2011 [15]. The 2012 Citizen Petition on metformin was followed by a systematic literature review on safety of metformin use among persons with mild to moderate renal insufficiency [16].

Sixth, drugs evaluated in the four Citizen Petitions had been initially approved by the FDA between 9 and 30 years previously. Safety concerns for thalidomide emerged three years after thalidomide received its 1996 FDA approval when clinical trials expanded thalidomide's use to the oncology setting. The approval was for cutaneous manifestations of leprosy. Identified ESA toxicities emerged after the initial FDA approval as clinical trials investigated off-label settings that evaluated longer durations of use and higher ESA doses- settings where unexpected toxicities emerged. The safety of metformin in the setting of mild to moderate renal insufficiency had been known for decades, but had not been reported in detail previously. Overall, the Petitions filled a void in the post-approved setting of drugs, where safety signals are frequently based on voluntary reports by clinicians to the FDA and manufacturers. Prior studies found that only 1% of serious reported adverse events are voluntarily reported, and the quality of these reports is generally low [17].

Policymakers have debated the timeliness and purpose of Citizen's Petitions, focusing on Citizen Petitions filed by pharmaceutical companies [18]. These Petitions seek to prevent market entry of generic competition, which account for 85% of filed Citizen Petitions with the FDA. Most Petitions filed by manufacturers of branded pharmaceuticals contain information that the Petitioner was aware of a long time prior to the filing of the Citizen Petition and that the primary purpose of the Petition was "last-ditch efforts" to delay generic competition. In contrast, the four successful Citizen Petitions were filed by individuals or non-profit organizations conducting health policy research related to patient safety (Tables 4.1 and 4.2). Two successful Citizen Petitions from health policy researchers requested revised Boxed Warnings for safety reasons for thalidomide, epoetin, and darbepoetin [19]. Two successful Citizen Petitions from health policy researchers requested liberalization of the Dosing section of the existing product label (Table 4.3) [11]. Each of the Citizen Petitions resulted in marked changes in practice. The thalidomide Citizen Petition heralded revised clinical guidelines that strongly recommended

Table 4.1 Research associated with four citizen petitions

	Thalidomide	Epoetin/Darbepoetin	Metformin	Metformin
Petitioner	Blumenthal	Cotter	Flory	Hennessey
Role	Conn AG	MTPPI-CEO	Yale	Penn
Request	Box warning	Box warning	Broader label	Same as Yale
Data support submitted in the Citizen Petition	Unpublished meta-analysis (Bennett)	Unpublished observational data base analysis (Cotter)	Unpublished systemic review (Flory)	Unpublished literature review (Hennessey)
Response date	2006	2011	2016	2016
Time to response	1 year	2 years	4 years	3 years
Funder for data analysis	R01	R01	K23, P30, K08	None listed
Data publication	JAMA 2006	Kidney International 2011	JAMA 2014	None listed

administration of venous thromboembolism prophylaxis (Table 4.5). The epoetin Citizen Petition heralded revised dosing guidelines for ESAs that removed trigger and target hemoglobin levels- and markedly reduced ESA use resulted (Tables 4.4 and 4.5). The metformin Citizen Petition allowed increased use of generic metformin by persons with mild to moderate renal insufficiency (Table 4.6).

4.2.1 Policy Implications

Our study reinforces the need to coordinate timely responses of pharmaceutical manufacturers and the FDA to Citizen Petitions requests that the FDA has granted in part or in full (Table 4.2). Going forward, it might be reasonable to require that the FDA respond to Citizen Petitions that request product label warnings or drug withdrawal for safety reasons within a 12-month time-period. While Congresspersons Rooney and Levin have sponsored STOP-GAMES legislation intended to decrease the number of frivolous Citizen Petitions filed by pharmaceutical manufacturers against competitors, we urge policymakers to consider introducing legislation that would facilitate timely review of Citizen Petitions and related response activities from health policy researchers who are conducting relevant policy research on pharmaceuticals or devices. This proposed legislation could be called Government Support of Clinical Information and Evaluation of Clinical Efficacy and Safety (GO-SCIENCES). It should be noted that the human and financial costs of one additional year of use of a "blockbuster" drug (i.e., a drug with $1 billion or more in annual sales) that has an unrecognized serious side effect are $8 billion in medical expenditures and 100,000 patients live affected by severe toxicity or death [1]. Thus, expediting Citizen Petition review and related safety activities within a 12-month period would have large clinical and financial implications.

Table 4.2 Researched associated with policy actions

	Thalidomide	Epoetin/Darbepoetin	Metformin	Metformin
Petitioner's Request	Box warning revision	Box warning revision	Use of eGFR as a measure of renal function	Use of eGFR as a measure of renal function
FDA action	Box warning revision	Warnings and precautions, dosing section revision	Revised warnings, precautions, and contraindications	Same
FDA data review	FDA meta-analysis	FDA review of clinical trial data, including trials reported after Petition was filed	FDA review of eGFR data that was not known at the time of the last label revision	Same
FDA conclusion of reason for partial granting of Petition	New safety information	New safety information	New safety information	Same
Grant number	1R01CA102713-01	R01-DK066011-01A2	None (Penn)	K23AG048359; (P30AG021342); K08HS023898 (Yale)
Manufacturer action: dear healthcare practitioner letter	2006	2011	Not done	Not done
FDA action: drug safety communication	None	2011	2016	2016
Manufacturer action: revised label and revised medication guide	2006	2011	2016	2016

Table 4.3 Summary of Label Changes for ESAs, Metformin, Thalidomide, and a thalidomide class-related agent (Revlimid)

ESA label changes (2011)
The ESA labels now **warn**:
• In <u>controlled trials</u> with CKD patients, patients experienced greater risks for death, serious adverse cardiovascular reactions, and stroke when administered ESAs to target a hemoglobin level of greater than 11 g/dL.
• No trial has identified a hemoglobin target level, ESA dose, or dosing strategy that does not increase these risks.
ESA labels now **recommend**:
• For patients with CKD, consider starting ESA treatment when the hemoglobin level is less than 10 g/dL. This advice does not define how far below 10 g/dL is appropriate for an individual to initiate. This advice also does not recommend that the goal is to achieve a hemoglobin of 10 g/dL or a hemoglobin dosing and use the lowest dose of ESA sufficient to reduce the need for red blood cell transfusions. Adjust dosing as appropriate
The drug label previously recommended that ESAs should be dosed to achieve and maintain hemoglobin levels within the target range of 10–12 g/dL in CKD patients. This target concept has been removed from the label.
Metformin Label Changes [August 2016]:
FDA is requiring manufacturers to revise the labeling of metformin-containing drugs to indicate that these products may be safely used in patients with mild to moderate renal impairment. See FDA Approved metformin-containing Medicines.
FDA is also requiring manufacturers to revise the labeling to recommend that the measure of kidney function used to determine whether a patient can receive metformin be changed from one based on a single laboratory parameter (blood creatinine concentration) to one that provides a better estimate of renal function (i.e., glomerular filtration rate estimating equation (eGFR)). This is because in addition to blood creatinine concentration, the glomerular filtration rate takes into account additional parameters that are important, such as the patient's age, gender, race, and/or weight. • The labeling recommendations on how and when kidney function is measured in patients receiving metformin will include the following information: • Before starting metformin, obtain the patient's eGFR. • Metformin is contra-indicated in patients with an eGFR below 30 mL/minute/1.73 m^2.
Starting metformin in patients with an eGFR between 30 and 45 mL/minute/1.73 m^2 is not recommended. • Obtain an eGFR at least annually in all patients taking metformin. In patients at increased risk for the development of renal impairment such as the elderly, renal function should be assessed more frequently. • In patients taking metformin whose eGFR later falls below 45 mL/minute/1.73 m^2, assess the benefits and risks of continuing treatment. Discontinue metformin if the patient's eGFR later falls below 30 mL/minute/1.73 m^2. • Discontinue metformin at the time of or before an iodinated contrast imaging procedure in patients with an eGFR between 30 and 60 mL/minute/1.73 m^2; in patients with a history of liver disease, alcoholism, or heart failure; or in patients who will be administered intra-arterial iodinated contrast. Reevaluate eGFR 48 h after the imaging procedure; restart metformin if renal function is stable
Thalidomide revised Boxed Warning [5/2006]:
Venous Thromboembolic Events: The use of Thalomid® (thalidomide) in multiple myeloma results in an increased risk of venous thromboembolic events, such as deep venous thrombosis and pulmonary embolus. This risk increases significantly when thalidomide is used in combination with standard chemotherapeutic agents including dexamethasone. In one controlled trial, the rate of venous thromboembolic events was 22.5% in patients receiving thalidomide in combination with dexamethasone compared to 4.9% in patients receiving dexamethasone alone (p = 0.002). Patients and physicians are advised to be observant for the signs and symptoms of thromboembolism. Patients should be instructed to seek medical care if they develop symptoms

(continued)

Table 4.3 (continued)

such as shortness of breath, chest pain, or arm or leg swelling. Preliminary data suggest that patients who are appropriate candidates may benefit from concurrent prophylactic anticoagulation or aspirin treatment.
Revlimid Boxed Warning (May 2006):
DEEP VENOUS THROMBOSIS AND PULMONARY EMBOLISM: This drug has demonstrated a significantly increased risk of deep venous thrombosis (DVT) and pulmonary embolism (PE) in patients with multiple myeloma who were treated with REVLIMID® (lenalidomide) combination therapy. Patients and physicians are advised to be observant for the signs and symptoms of thromboembolism. Patients should be instructed to seek medical care if they develop symptoms such as shortness of breath, chest pain, or arm or leg swelling. It is not known whether prophylactic anticoagulation or antiplatelet therapy prescribed in conjunction with REVLIMID® 139 (lenalidomide) may lessen the potential for venous thromboembolic events. The decision to take prophylactic measures should be done carefully after an assessment of an individual patient's underlying risk factors.

Table 4.4 Summary of medication guide changes

Thalidomide—Medication Guide Changes Resulting from Citizen Petition
Blood clots. People with multiple myeloma (MM) who take THALOMID may have an increased risk for blood clots in their arteries, veins, and lungs. This risk is even higher if you take the medicine dexamethasone with THALOMID to treat your MM. Heart attacks and strokes may also happen if you take THALOMID with dexamethasone.
Epoetin and Darbepoetin—Medication Guide Changes Resulting from Citizen Petition
For all patients who take PROCRIT, ARANESP, OR EPOGEN, including patients with cancer or chronic kidney disease: • If you decide to take PROCRIT, ARANESP, OR EPOGEN, your healthcare provider should prescribe.
Revlimid Medication Guide Changes (May 2006):
• REVLIMID may cause serious side effects including:
Blood clots. Blood clots in the arteries, veins, and lungs happen more often in people who take REVLIMID. This risk is even higher for people with multiple myeloma who take the medicine dexamethasone with REVLIMID. Heart attacks and strokes also happen more often in people who take REVLIMID with dexamethasone.

Table of Key Trials for ESAs in CKD

Administrative and correspondence documents for Application 21-430 (thalidomide as a treatment for multiple myeloma) US Food and Drug Administration, Center for Drug Evaluation and Research http://www.accessdata.fda.gov/drugsatfda_docs/nda/2006/021430s000_AdminCorres.pdf

Sources of Funding for each of the Citizen Petitions

Metformin: Dr. Lipska received support from the National Institute on Aging and the American Federation of Aging Research through the Paul Beeson Career Development Award (K23AG048359) and the Yale Claude D. Pepper Older Americans Independence Center (P30AG021342). Dr. Flory received support from the Agency for Healthcare Research and Quality through a career development award (K08HS023898).

Table 4.5 Thalidomide post-marketing commitments that resulted from the citizen petition (May 2006)

As a condition of FDA granting accelerated approval for thalidomide as a treatment for multiple myeloma, the manufacturer was required to:
Conduct an epidemiologic study (An Epidemiology Study of Venous Thrombotic Events in Thalidomide Treated Multiple Myeloma Patients) to address the questions detailed below:
Safety questions:
1. What is the failure rate for each of the different types of thromboembolic prophylaxis (e.g., antiplatelet or anticoagulant therapy) for MM patients treated with a thalidomide-containing regimen?
2. What is the failure rate for each type of DVT treatment (dose-adjusted heparin, low molecular weight heparin, coumadin) for those patients with MM and a DVT who continue to receive ongoing treatment with thalidomide?
3. What is the failure rate for each type of post-DVT thromboembolic prophylaxis for those patients with MM and a DVT who continue to receive ongoing treatment with thalidomide? This prospective epidemiologic study will enroll select patients identified in the S.T.E.P.S. program, and collect the necessary additional data on these patients to further evaluate occurrences of thrombosis and anticoagulant use. The final details of the design will be as agreed between the Agency and Celgene. The dates for submission of the protocol, study start date and final report submission are indicated below: NDA 21-430 NDA 20-785/S-031 Page 3 Protocol Submission: October 2006 Study Start: March 2007 Final Report Submission: March 2010.

Table 4.6 Summary of lenalidomide safety initiatives (May 2006)

We [The FDA] also remind you of your post-marketing study commitments specified in your submission dated June 26, 2006. These commitments, along with any completion dates agreed upon, are listed below
A. Conduct an epidemiologic study to address the questions detailed below:
1. What is the failure rate for each of the different types of thromboembolic prophylaxis (e.g., antiplatelet or anticoagulant therapy) for multiple myeloma patients treated with a lenalidomide containing regimen?
2. What is the failure rate for each type of Deep Vein Thrombosis (DVT) treatment (dose-adjusted heparin, low molecular weight heparin, coumadin) for those patients with multiple myeloma and a DVT who continue to receive ongoing treatment with lenalidomide?
3. What is the failure rate for each type of post-DVT thromboembolic prophylaxis for those patients with multiple myeloma and a DVT who continue to receive ongoing treatment with lenalidomide? NDA 21-880/S-001 Page 2 This prospective epidemiologic study will enroll select patients identified in the RevAssistSM program, and collect the necessary additional data on these patients to further evaluate occurrences of thrombosis and anticoagulant use. The final details of the design will be as agreed upon between the Agency and Celgene. Protocol Submission: by December 2006 Study Start: by June 2007 Final Report Submission: by December 2012.

Thalidomide: Dr. Bennett received support from the Centers for Economic Excellence Program of the State of South Carolina, the Doris Meddin Levkoff Center for Medication Safety, Grants No. 1R01CA102713-01 from the National Cancer Institute., and

Epoetin: Dr. Cotter was supported in part by National Institutes of above 10 g/dL. Individualize Health grant R01-DK066011-01A2.

References

1. Bennett CL, Angelotta C, Yarnold PR et al (2006) Thalidomide- and lenalidomide-associated thromboembolism among patients with cancer. JAMA 296:2558–2560
2. Chen BK, Yang YT, Cheng X, Bian J, Bennett CL (2016) Petitioning the FDA to improve pharmaceutical, device and public health safety by ordinary citizens: a descriptive analysis. PLoS ONE 11:e0155259
3. Chen B, Restaino J, Norris L, Xirasagar S, Qureshi ZP, McKoy JM, et al (2012) A Tale of two citizens: a state attorney general and a hematologist facilitate translation of research into US food and drug administration actions—a sonar report. J Oncol Pract. JOP.2011.000504
4. Feldman R, Wang C (2017) A citizen's petition process gone astray. Delaying competition from generic drugs. N Engl J Med 376:1499–1501. https://doi.org/10.1056/NEJMp1700202
5. Lipska KJ, Flory JH, Hennessy S, Inzucchi SE (2016) Citizen petition to the US food and drug administration to change prescribing guidelines: the metformin experience. Circulation 134:1405–1408
6. FDA/CDER Response to Connecticut attorney general's office—partial approval/denial letter
7. FDA/CDER Response to Illinois attorney general's office and public citizen health research group—partial approval/denial letter
8. Thamer M, Zhang Y, Kaufman J, Cotter D, Dong F, Hernán MA (2007) Dialysis facility ownership and epoetin dosing in patients receiving hemodialysis. JAMA 297(15):1667–1674
9. HR 2387, the Stop the Overuse of Petitions and Get Affordable Medicines to Enter Soon (STOP GAMES) Act of 2019. Sponsored by Andy Levin (D-Michigan) and Francis Rooney R-Florida)
10. Regulations.gov. University of Pennsylvania and Cornell University Petition. Citizen Petition to revise the label of Metformin
11. Woodcock J. Director, FDA Center for drug evaluation and research. Response to Citizen Petition FDA-2009-P-0246 for Label Change for Epogen®. June 24, 2011
12. Citizen petitions, 21 code of federal regulations 10.30
13. FDA Drug Safety Communication: Modified dosing recommendations to improve the safe use of Erythropoiesis-Stimulating Agents (ESAs) in chronic kidney disease. June 24, 2011
14. FDA Drug Safety Podcast for Healthcare Professionals: Modified dosing recommendations to improve the safe use of Erythropoiesis-Stimulating Agents (ESAs) in chronic kidney disease
15. Woodcock J. Letter to Dr. Charles L. Bennett (re FDA-P-2014-1611). University of South Carolina. July 10, 2018
16. Inzucchi SE, Lipska KJ, Mayo H, Bailey CJ, McGuire DK (2014) Metformin in patients with type 2 diabetes and kidney disease: a systematic review. JAMA 312:2668–2675
17. Moore TJ, Bennett CL (2012) Underreporting of hemorrhagic and thrombotic complications of pharmaceuticals to the U.S. Food and Drug Administration: empirical findings for warfarin, clopidogrel, ticlopidine, and thalidomide from the Southern Network on Adverse Reactions (SONAR). Semin Thromb Hemost 38(8):905–7
18. Carrier MA, Wander D (2012) Citizen petitions: an empirical study. Cardozo L Rev. 34:249
19. Citizen petition to the FDA for label change to FQ label to include psychiatric toxicities. Filed 9/9/2013 and posted 10/1/2014 as FDA-2014-P-1611-0001

Paul Ray DO. FACOS is an Adjunct Professor University of South Carolina and a Clinical Adjunct Professor at Midwestern University in Downers Grove, Illinois. Dr. Ray received his master's degree based on research studying the protective mechanism action of taurine on ouabain infusions on the dog heart. This was his first publication in medical school, which he completed in 3 years and was also in the top 10 percent of his class. He continued publishing during his Urology residency at the University of Illinois. He became the second Osteopath admitted to any Allopathic Urology Residency program and to become Board Certified by the American Board of Urology. Shortly after finishing his Residency, he was appointed Chairman of Urology at Cook County Hospital.

Charles L. Bennett MD, Ph.D. MPP, SmartState Chair and Frank P. and Josie M. Fletcher Chair of Medication Safety and Efficacy and Director, SmartState Center for Medication Safety and Efficacy, is also a Visiting Scholar at the City of Hope National Cancer Institute Designated Comprehensive Cancer Center in Duarte, California and is the co-editor of this book, Cancer Policy (2nd Edition). Dr. Bennett is a Phi Beta Kappa and High Honors graduate in mathematics from Swarthmore College, earned his medical degree in 1981 from the University of Pennsylvania Perelman School of Medicine, and completed internal medicine, hematology, and oncology training at the Michael Reese Hospital and the University of Chicago Pritzger School of Medicine before completing his Ph.D. and Masters In Public Policy degrees with honors in social science at the RAND Pardee Graduate School of Public Policy in Santa Monica, California. He has led a 20-year National Institutes of Health funded pharmacovigilance called the Research on Adverse Drug events And Reports (RADAR) and subsequently called to Southern Network on Adverse drug Reactions (SONAR) at the University of South Carolina College of Pharmacy.

Systemic Barriers and Potential Concerns from Reporting Serious Adverse Drug Reactions

5

Matthew A. Taylor, Ashley C. Godwin, Shamia Hoque, and Charles L. Bennett

5.1 Introduction

About 1–10% of all serious adverse drug reactions (sADRs) are reported to the Food and Drug Administration (FDA) [1]. Prevailing opinion suggests that low reporting rates reflect time constraints. Even when possible ADRs are reported, the reporting quality is poor [2]. While investigating fifty sADRs over the past two decades as Principal Investigator of the largest publicly funded adverse event watchdog group (RADAR/SONAR), [CLB] encountered several physicians who communicated personal concerns when reporting sADRs to the FDA or pharmaceutical regulatory agencies in other countries. In nine instances, the physician had reported a sADR that subsequently was associated with a Black Box warning or drug withdrawal from market [3, 4]. Interestingly, none of their concerns with reporting involved time constraints. These ADR experiences provide context for understanding reasons why physicians rarely report ADRs. In each instance, the related sADR resulted in a serious outcome, including organ transplantation, serious organ failure, or death. Individual experiences from clinical investigators were reviewed for information on personal barriers to clinician sADR reporting.

M. A. Taylor · A. C. Godwin · S. Hoque · C. L. Bennett (✉)
SONAR (Southern Network on Adverse Reactions) Program, University of South Carolina Colleges of Pharmacy and Engineering, Columbia, SC 29208, USA
e-mail: bennettc@cop.sc.edu

M. A. Taylor
e-mail: matthew_taylor@brown.edu

A. C. Godwin
e-mail: godwina@email.sc.edu

S. Hoque
e-mail: hoques@cec.sc.edu

Table 5.1 summarizes the consequences and is elaborated in the next sections. This project received Institutional Review Board approval from the University of South Carolina.

Table 5.1 Summary of nine reasons and consequences of reporting sADRs

Main factor		Event
Litigation Risk	1. Fear of being included in a lawsuit against the manufacture	1. Patient died from PML; family filed lawsuit; physician included as defendant
	2. Fear of being sued for libel	2. Gadodiamide reported as most likely cause of NSF; manufacturer-initiated libel suit
	3. Fear of personally sued for malpractice	3. Physician prescribed nevirapine and was concerned that the hepatotoxicity developed by patient was an sADR but did not report it to FDA
	4. Fear of physician partners being sued for malpractice	4. Physician reported adverse effects of power morcellator procedure when the statute of limitations passed
Professional Retaliation	1. Fear of exclusion from cooperative industry—sponsored clinical trials	1. Clinician hesitant to report a case of a patient's death from PML following treatment with a novel drug due to concerns that he or she will not be included in phase III clinical trials
	2. Fear of jeopardizing existing academic collaborations	2. Cardiologist did not report an event to the FDA for fear that it will negatively impact ongoing collaborations with other academic investigators and ties to the manufacturer
	3 Fear of being excluded from a pharmaceutical corporation's speaker's bureau	3. Clinician concerned that the pharmaceutical manufacturer might not include him or her as a future speaker in pharmaceutical sponsored lecture series
Regulatory Consideration	1. Concern that no response from FDA was likely	1. Clinician was uncertain that a causal relationship existed between a drug and the adverse reaction and did thought reporting to FDA will have any meaningful results
	2. Concern that no response from the FDA was needed	2. Oncologist noted that the sADR was already noted in the product label and did not report

This table provides a summary of the nine physician experiences with sADRs as described throughout the manuscript text. The experiences are divided into three categories based on the nature of their primary concern: Legal, Professional, or Regulatory (left column). The primary concern with reporting is described (middle column) and a brief summary of the events involved with the case is shown (right column)

5.2   Findings of Litigation Risks

5.2.1   Fear of Being Included in a Lawsuit Against the Manufacturer

At a medical conference, a clinician reported personally to the RADAR Principal Investigator details involving a child undergoing off-label Rituximab therapy for Immune Thrombocytopenia Purpura (ITP). The child then presented with Progressive Multifocal Leukoencephalopathy (PML), a rare fatal central nervous system infection caused by the John Cunningham (JC) virus. Rituximab-associated PML was previously reported by RADAR in 2006 among 57 patients with non-Hodgkin's lymphoma. Those cases occurred following treatment with a novel monoclonal Ibritumomab treatment, and among Rituximab-treated persons with Rheumatoid Arthritis or Crohn's disease [5]. De-identified information about this patient was reported by RADAR to the FDA in an effort to improve the public health and the public safety of Rituximab. Unfortunately, the child in this case soon died from PML. One year later, the patient's family filed a lawsuit with the manufacturer of Rituximab stating that the PML safety concerns had not been fully explained in Rituximab's product label. The lawsuit included the physician who initially reported the case to RADAR as a defendant. After the physician was deposed by lawyers representing the manufacturer, the physician was dropped from the lawsuit. The patient's family and the manufacturer negotiated an undisclosed settlement.

5.2.2   Fear of Being Sued for Libel

In 2012, the chairman of a large hospital in Denmark communicated personal experiences when reporting the first cases of a previously unrecognized sADR, termed Gadodiamide-associated Nephrogenic Systemic Fibrosis (NSF) [6]. This sADR is a dermatologic and systemic fibrosis that occurs rapidly after administration of linear chelated Gadolinium-based contrast agents that is administered to persons with chronic kidney disease or persons with acute kidney injury who are undergoing MRI scans. While NSF was initially discovered among 5 patients in one Austrian hospital in 2006, the linear chelated Gadolinium-based contrast agent [Gadodiamide] was identified as the probable cause of the toxicity. After two years of evaluation, it was discovered that 1,500 persons in 50 hospitals in the United States, 64 persons in eight hospitals in Denmark, and 30 persons in hospitals in other countries had also developed NSF.

In 2007, the Danish radiologist and a collaborating nephrologist from the same hospital were the first to publish that Gadodiamide was the most likely cause [7]. These clinicians had reported the sADR information to the country's Ministry of Health in 2006 [6]. In 2008, the radiologist described Gadodiamide as the proximate cause of NSF at a medical conference at Oxford University. The manufacturer then initiated a libel lawsuit against the radiologist who had identified the association between a single product and NSF. Subsequently, at a courtroom trial involving Gadodiamide's manufacturer and a NSF patient, attorneys for the plaintiff presented a 1993 unpublished document that showed the manufacturer's scientists had reported high levels of free Gadolinium in anephric rats following Gadodiamide administration [8, 9]. One day later, both lawsuits were dropped and settlement agreements were reached [10]. The reporting physician was placed on academic leave for one year but was eventually reinstated to his previously held position. Between 2011 and 2014, the manufacturer settled hundreds of individual law suits with CKD patients who had developed NSF following Gadodiamide administration. The manufacturer had lost only three Gadodiamide-associated NSF cases at a mass tort trial [11].

5.2.3 Fear of Personally Being Sued for Malpractice

A physician at an occupational health department prescribed two weeks of an HIV-drug, Nevirapine, for post-exposure prophylaxis (PEP) to a nurse who had experienced a needle stick exposure from fluids from an HIV-infected patient during a procedure. After the nurse completed the two-week PEP regimen, she developed severe hepatotoxicity that resolved after several months of high dose corticosteroids [12]. The occupational health physician who had prescribed the Nevirapine was concerned that sADR reporting might facilitate a malpractice lawsuit from the patient. The physician was uncertain that Nevirapine was the primary cause of hepatitis and reported case details to RADAR. RADAR in turn reported case details (with personal information deidentification) to FDA's Med-Watch Program, the Centers for Disease Control and Protection, the safety department of Nevirapine's manufacturer, and in two publications [12, 13]. Concurrently, a public health physician in London reported five HIV-exposed women had developed severe hepatitis within days of receiving Nevirapine-containing PEP after being sexually assaulted [14]. Three physicians from the safety program asked the reporting physician if he could review the FDA report to indicate that the toxicity was "associated with the drug, but not caused by the drug". Shortly thereafter, the infectious disease physician left their home institution and now practices at a neighboring hospital.

5.2.4 Fear of Physician Partners Being Sued for Malpractice

The RADAR PI was contacted by a cardiothoracic surgeon about a sADR involving his wife, also a physician. This patient had undergone a power morcellator procedure to remove a uterine fibroid and subsequently died from metastatic uterine sarcoma [Narchasm H, Personal Communication]. The treating gynecologist had reported previously that another woman had undergone a fibroidectomy with a power morcellator at the same medical center and had died just prior to his wife's procedure [15]. The husband reported to the FDA details of his wife's case. This led to FDA requiring that the manufacturer issue warnings against power morcellator use, a label change, and ultimately withdrawal from the market. A 2017 Government Accountability Organization report identified a 1 in 350 cancer risk in fibroids and highlighted three cases of fatal metastatic sarcoma developing among women who had undergone power morcellator procedure years earlier [16]. A physician, concerned that reporting these cases might lead to malpractice lawsuits, reported the adverse events to the FDA only after the statute of limitations had passed. In 2014, the FDA and several insurers withdrew support for morcellator procedures after identifying hundreds of women worldwide who had developed uterine sarcoma following power morcellator.

5.3   Professional Retaliation

5.3.1   Fear of Exclusion from Cooperative Industry-Sponsored Clinical Trials

A clinician reported to the SONAR PI details of a patient who died from PML following off-label treatment outside of a clinical trial of a novel immunoconjugate that the FDA had approved for lymphoma. The patient had received three doses of the bio-drug conjugate. The clinician was hesitant to report the case to the manufacturer because causality was uncertain and there was concern the physician might not be included as a co-investigator for a phase III clinical trial studying a new clinical indication of the drug. The clinician was not selected to participate in this trial; however, after some months had passed, they were chosen to participate in another multi-institutional study. The SONAR PI reported de-identified information on the case to the FDA after personally redacting information on the physician, hospital, and city. A revised boxed warning describing PML and the drug was subsequently added to the product label, although a causal rationale was listed as uncertain.

5.3.2   Fear of Jeopardizing Existing Academic Collaborations

An interventional cardiologist placed a drug eluting stent into the coronary artery of a patient with a narrow coronary artery. Two weeks later the patient died and an autopsy identified an eosinophilic infiltrate at the site of the stent. The cardiologist informed the RADAR PI that this event was not reported to the FDA as a possible adverse device event because of concern that this might jeopardize ongoing collaborations with other academic investigators with strong ties to the manufacturer. The RADAR PI reported de-identified clinical findings to FDA's MedWatch Program. The cardiologist and co-investigators published clinical findings of four cases that included autopsy findings and 12 additional cases that did not have autopsy findings. The FDA issued a Public Health notification about allergic reactions to drug eluting stents, and then withdrew the notification one month later [17, 18].

5.3.3 Fear of Being Excluded from a Pharmaceutical Corporation's Speaker's Bureau

An oncologist treated a breast cancer patient with a supportive care pharmaceutical following four cycles of chemotherapy. Three months after initiating this therapy, the patient developed a fatal pulmonary embolism. The oncologist was aware that the product label had been recently revised to include a boxed warning related to drug-associated venous thromboembolism. The oncologist informed RADAR that details of this case was not reported to the FDA or to the manufacturer as a causal relationship was uncertain, the toxicity had recently been added to the product label, and there was concern that the pharmaceutical manufacturer might not include the clinician as a speaker in future pharmaceutical sponsored lecture series. In 2008, RADAR reported a meta-analysis identifying 1.57-fold increased risks for epoetin-associated venous thromboembolism [19].

5.4 Regulatory Considerations

5.4.1 Concern that no Response from the FDA Was Likely

A clinician provider of therapeutic apheresis services identified a patient who was undergoing treatment for Thrombotic Thrombocytopenic Purpura (TTP). The patient had been prescribed Ticlopidine two weeks prior to the TTP onset. The clinician expressed concern that a causal relationship between Ticlopidine and TTP was certain and that reporting this information to the FDA should result in meaningful safety practices. RADAR and others described 59 cases of TPP following Ticlopidine use, and the FDA subsequently issued a Black Box Warning related to the sADR one year later [20]. Because of safety concerns and the FDA approval of a safer medication, sales of Ticlopidine in the United States ceased. Because of the low price of generics, Ticlopidine is still commonly prescribed in Japan and Ticlopidine-associated TTP still occurs in Japan [21].

5.4.2 Concern that no Response from the FDA Was Needed

An oncologist treated an elderly patient with non-Hodgkin's lymphoma with a Rituximab-containing chemotherapy regimen. Several months after initiating this treatment, the patient developed PML and died. The oncologist was aware that the product label had been revised to identify six cases of Rituximab and PML (although a causal pathway had not been reported). The oncologist reported the case of Rituximab-associated PML to the RADAR PI, stating that this adverse drug reaction was already well-described in the revised product label. RADAR and collaborators reported this case and 56 additional cases of Rituximab-associated PML and a Black Box warning describing this toxicity was added to the product label [5]. Senior officials from the manufacturer met with the RADAR PI and requested that the word "association" replace the word "causal" in the adverse event report.

5.5 Discussion

Physicians rarely report sADRs to the FDA. The most commonly cited reason is being too busy. Other reasons include litigation, reprisals, and uncertainty that this information is useful to regulatory agencies. Physicians are also concerned that reporting potential ADRs can have negative personal and professional consequences. It is worth noting that patients do not realize the obstacles physicians often face in reporting sADRs.

Our findings have important implications. While anonymity of reporting physicians is assured in theory, this may not happen in practice. In one instance where sADRs were reported to the manufacturers' safety department, representatives from the manufacturer visited the reporting physician to request additional clinical information and to request a revision of the semantics of the report.

Legal and economic implications must be considered. Physicians who report sADRs must receive legal protection from the patients affected by the related toxicity. The hesitancy of surgeons at one hospital to report metastatic sarcoma development after power morcellator procedures until the statute of limitations had passed is disconcerting. In response to this reporting failure, some policymakers are recommending that physicians who fail to communicate serious ADR information to the FDA may be at risk for personal lawsuits or criminal charges. Economically, sADRs contribute to increased cost in physician malpractice insurance; thus, raising the overall cost of healthcare [22]. A short-sided and undesirable solution to this cost concern is not to report and identify sADRs, which may save money, but to the detriment of patient safety.

Professionalism is another consideration. Overarching government body interference with a physician's medical practice can cause unwanted complications and time constraints. A patient developing a sADR shortly after a prescribed therapy can be devastating to the physician. Reporting the event voluntarily to the FDA, hospital, or pharmaceutical manufacturer may not occur, because of concern over personal liability. Clinical practice settings should offer collegial support to facilitate physician reporting of ADRs in these settings.

Several long-term solutions exist. Increased funding of pharmacovigilance centers that prospectively seek to identify important ADRs should be considered. Another option would be to develop electronic reporting systems that could be readily accessed by smartphones and other devices, while maintaining patient confidentiality. Regulators and insurers should consider allowing physicians to bill for time spent reporting ADRs. These reports must be easily completed, yet include comprehensive information on sociodemographics, comorbidities, drug doses & duration of use, other concomitant drugs, diagnostic tests, and patient outcome. Currently, only 20–50% of these elements are included in ADR reports submitted by pharmaceutical manufacturers to the FDA or by clinicians to an IRB [23, 24]. Some policy initiatives in the United States and Canada urge that reporting should be compulsory for "suspected" ADRs and suspected Adverse Device Reactions [25, 26]. While this would be infeasible for all ADRs, certain sentinel events might be developed—such as hepatic failure, hemolytic uremic syndrome, TTP, suicide, neuropsychiatric toxicity, and severe anaphylaxis.

The Citizen Process was used by attorneys and separately by clinicians to provide contrasting recommendations to the FDA related to gadolinium-based contrast agents. Over 95% of Citizen Petition's filed with the FDA are submitted by representatives of pharmaceutical manufacturers who are protesting against their competitors, rather than by patients, patient families, or attorneys who represent patients. A concern by attorneys representing patients is that if the Petition is denied, it can adversely affect subsequent litigation by excluding certain potentially causal factors. In this instance, the Petition was ruled on favorably in part and denied in part- but overall assisted with the tort litigation. An average of two Petitions annually by citizens are ruled on favorably by the FDA. One safety-related Citizen Petition filed in 2005 by the RADAR PI in conjunction with then Connecticut Attorney General Richard Blumenthal was ruled as granted in part and denied in part by the FDA in 2006. A second Citizen Petition was filed by the SONAR PI in September 2014 and received a decision on July 10, 2018; almost four years later. The concern expressed in the Petition was reviewed in 2015 by an FDA Advisory Committee where votes of 20–1, 18–0, and 19–2 in favor of the Petition were recorded, and requested changes in the Product Label have been partially completed [24, 27]. Citizen Petitions, when used appropriately, may be another avenue for sADR reporting (Table 5.1).

Pharmaceutical safety and reporting of ADRs will be increasingly challenging since passage of the 21st Century Cures Act. Emphasis has been placed on shortening the time to FDA approval of new drugs [28]. While ADR reporting may serve as an important safety effort in the future, barriers to ADR reporting identified herein will need to be addressed if improvements in the quality and number of physician ADR reports are to occur.

References

1. Moore T, Bennett C (2012) Underreporting of hemorrhagic and thrombotic complications of pharmaceuticals to the U.S. Food and Drug Administration: empirical findings for warfarin, clopidogrel, ticlopidine, and thalidomide from the southern network on adverse reactions (SONAR). Semin Thromb Hemost 38(08):905–907. https://doi.org/10.1055/s-0032-1328890

2. Dorr DA, Burdon R, West DP et al (2009) Quality of reporting of serious adverse drug events to an institutional review board: a case study with the novel cancer agent Imatinib Mesylate. Clin Cancer Res 15(11):3850–3855. https://doi.org/10.1158/1078-0432.CCR-08-1811

3. Lu K, Kessler S, Schulz R, et al (2014) Systematic Approach to Pharmacovigilance beyond the Limits: the southern network on adverse reactions (SONAR) Projects. Adv Pharmacoepidemiol Drug Saf 3(2). https://doi.org/10.4172/2167-1052.1000149

4. Bennett CL, Nebeker JR, Lyons EA et al (2005) The research on adverse drug events and reports (RADAR) project. JAMA 293(17):2131–2140. https://doi.org/10.1001/jama.293.17.2131

5. Carson KR, Evens AM, Richey EA et al (2009) Progressive multifocal leukoencephalopathy after rituximab therapy in HIV-negative patients: a report of 57 cases from the Research on Adverse Drug Events and Reports project. Blood 113(20):4834–4840. https://doi.org/10.1182/blood-2008-10-186999

6. Bennett CL, Starko KM, Thomsen HS, et al (2012) Linking drugs to obscure illnesses: lessons from pure red cell aplasia, nephrogenic systemic fibrosis, and Reye's syndrome. a report from the Southern Network on Adverse Reactions (SONAR). J Gen Intern Med 27(12):1697–1703. https://doi.org/10.1007/s11606-012-2098-1

7. Marckmann P, Skov L, Rossen K et al (2006) Nephrogenic systemic fibrosis: suspected causative role of gadodiamide used for contrast-enhanced magnetic resonance imaging. J Am Soc Nephrol 17(9):2359–2362. https://doi.org/10.1681/ASN.2006060601

8. United States Court of Appeals SC .(2014) Decker V. GE Healthcare Inc GE AS. No. 13-400. https://caselaw.findlaw.com/us-6th-circuit/1681196.html.

9. Travis J (2009) MRI drug debate sparks libel suit against scientist. Sci Mag. https://www.sciencemag.org/news/2009/12/mri-drug-debate-sparks-libel-suit-against-scientist. Published December 2009. Accessed 9 Feb 2018

10. Wogan T (2010) Facing own lawsuit, firm drops libel suit against researcher. Sci Mag. https://www.sciencemag.org/news/2010/02/facing-own-lawsuit-firm-drops-libel-suit-against-researcher. Published 2010. Accessed 9 Feb 2018

11. $5 Million verdict in gadolinium case upheld by US court of appeals. https://ashcraftandgerel.com/news/5-million-verdict-in-gadolinium-case-upheld-by-u-s-court-of-appeals/. Accessed 9 Feb 2018

12. Johnson S, Baraboutis JG (2000) Adverse effects associated with use of nevirapine in HIV postexposure prophylaxis for 2 health care workers. JAMA 284(21):2722–2723. https://doi.org/10.1001/jama.284.21.2717

13. Johnson S, Chan J, Bennett CL (2002) Hepatotoxicity after prophylaxis with a nevirapine-containing antiretroviral regimen. Ann Intern Med 137(2):146. https://doi.org/10.7326/0003-4819-137-2-200207160-00025

14. Benn PD, Mercey DE, Brink N, Scott G, Williams IG (2001) Prophylaxis with a nevirapine-containing triple regimen after exposure to HIV-1. Lancet 357(9257):687–688. https://doi.org/10.1016/S0140-6736(00)04139-8

15. Hingston S (2016) What are the chances? A tale of love vs. big medicine. Phila Mag. https://www.phillymag.com/news/2016/03/20/amy-reed-morcellation/. Published 2016. Accessed 9 Feb 2018

16. Requesters GR to C. Medical devices: cancer risk led to warn against certain uses of power morcellators and recommend new labeling. 2017. https://www.gao.gov/assets/690/682573.pdf

17. Administration F and D. Information for Physicians on Sub-Acute Thromboses (SAT) and Hypersensitivity Reactions with Use of the Cordis CYPHER Coronary Stent. FDA Public Health Web Notification (1st Edition)
18. Administration F and D. Updated Information for Physicians on Sub-acute Thromboses (SAT) and Hypersensitivity Reactions with Use of the Cordis CYPHER Sirolimus-eluting Coronary Stent. FDA Public Health Web Notification (1st Edition)
19. Bennett CL, Angelotta C, Yarnold PR et al (2006) thalidomide- and lenalidomide-associated thromboembolism among patients with cancer. JAMA 296(21):2555. https://doi.org/10.1001/jama.296.21.2558-c
20. Bennett CL, Weinberg PD, Rozenberg-Ben-Dror K, Yarnold PR, Kwaan HC, Green D (1998) Thrombotic thrombocytopenic purpura associated with ticlopidine. A review of 60 cases. Ann Intern Med 128(7):541–544. https://doi.org/10.7326/0003-4819-128-7-199804010-00004
21. Bennett CL, Jacob S, Dunn BL et al (2013) Ticlopidine-associated ADAMTS13 activity deficient thrombotic thrombocytopenic purpura in 22 persons in Japan: a report from the Southern Network on Adverse Reactions (SONAR). Br J Haematol 161(6):896–898. https://doi.org/10.1111/bjh.12303
22. Frakes M, Gruber J (2018) Defensive medicine: evidence from military immunity. Cambridge, MA. https://doi.org/10.3386/w24846
23. Bennett CL, Nebeker JR, Yarnold PR et al (2007) Evaluation of serious adverse drug reactions: a proactive pharmacovigilance program (RADAR) vs safety activities conducted by the Food and Drug Administration and pharmaceutical manufacturers. Arch Intern Med 167 (10):1041–1049. https://doi.org/10.1001/archinte.167.10.1041
24. Moore TJ, Furberg CD, Mattison DR, Cohen MR (2016) Completeness of serious adverse drug event reports received by the US Food and Drug Administration in 2014. Pharmacoepidemiol Drug Saf 25(6):713–718. https://doi.org/10.1002/pds.3979
25. Fitzpatrick BK (2017) Medical device guardians act. In: 115th congress:H.R.2163. https://www.congress.gov/bill/115th-congress/house-bill/2163
26. Protecting Canadians from Unsafe Drugs Act (Vanessa's Law). Second Session, Forty-First Parliament (2018). http://www.parl.ca/DocumentViewer/en/41-2/bill/C-17/royal-assent.
27. J Woodcock (2018) Re . Docket No. FDA-2014-P-1611. (Received from Janet Woodcock by Charles L. Bennett on 10 July 2018)
28. Knopf K, Baum M, Shimp WS et al (2016) Interpretation of surrogate endpoints in the era of the 21st century cures act. BMJ 355:i6286. https://doi.org/10.1136/bmj.i6286

Matthew A. Taylor MD, MS is a first-year resident at the Brown University School of Medicine internal medicine program in Providence, Rhode Island. He has been an active collaborator under the guidance of Shamia Hoque, Ph.D. and Charles L Bennett, MD, Ph.D., MPP in the SONAR projects efforts to develop novel approaches to understanding adverse drug reactions.

Ashley C. Godwin Ph.D. is a recent graduate of the University of South Carolina's College of Pharmacy Clinical Pharmacy and Outcomes Studies (CPOS) Ph.D. program. She has presented SONAR findings at poster presentations at the American Society of Clinical Oncology's annual conferences.

Shamia Hoque Ph.D., Associate Professor, Department of Civil Engineering, University of South Carolina and Principal Investigator for the American Cancer Society Institutional Research Grant on novel analytic approaches to identifying adverse drug reactions. She is a long-term co-investigator with Dr. Bennett and the SONAR project.

Charles L. Bennett MD, Ph.D., MPP, SmartState Chair and Frank P and Josie M Fletcher Chair of Medication Safety and Efficacy and Director, SmartState Center for Medication Safety and Efficacy, is also a Visiting Scholar at the City of Hope National Cancer Institute Designated Comprehensive Cancer Center in Duarte, California and is the co-editor of this book, Cancer Policy (2nd Edition). Dr. Bennett is a Phi Beta Kappa and High Honors graduate in mathematics from Swarthmore College, earned his medical degree in 1981 from the University of Pennsylvania Perelman School of Medicine, and completed internal medicine, hematology, and oncology training at the Michael Reese Hospital and the University of Chicago Pritzger School of Medicine before completing his Ph.D. and Masters In Public Policy degrees with honors in social science at the RAND Pardee Graduate School of Public Policy in Santa Monica, California. He has led a 20-year National Institutes of Health funded pharmacovigilance called the Research on Adverse Drug events And Reports (RADAR) and subsequently called to Southern Network on Adverse drug Reactions (SONAR) at the University of South Carolina College of Pharmacy.

Was There Something Rotten in Denmark: Nephrogenic System Fibrosis Cases Occurring in Copenhagen

6

Charles L. Bennett, Bartlett Witherspoon, Kenneth R. Carson, and Henrik S. Thomsen

6.1 Introduction

More than half of all serious adverse drug reactions are identified seven years after FDA approval [1]. One recent and unusual example involves a syndrome initially termed nephrogenic dermatopathic fibrosis, and then called nephrogenic systemic fibrosis (NSF) [2]. It is a rare disorder characterized by skin changes that mimic progressive localized systemic sclerosis. The disorder as characterized in 2007 by the Food and Drug Administration in the United States and in 2008 by the Danish Medicines Agency was associated with administration of two specific brands of gadolinium-based contrast agents (GBCAs) to persons with chronic kidney disease (CKD) [3, 4]. These patients had undergone magnetic resonance (MR) imaging procedures at a Herlev Hospital,a large hospital in Copenhagen during 2003 to 2006. Denmark, with a population of 5.5 million persons, is an international leader in identifying and evaluating NSF. This chapter reviews why the Danish experience was the second to be identified in the world in 2006 and one of the first to eradicated this this rare illness by 2008. Such rapid eradication of what was shortly identified as a world wide "epidemic" is distinctly unusual (Table 6.2).

Seven formulations of GBCAs have been approved by the European Medicines Agency and/or the Danish Medicines Agency (Table 6.1) [4]. In 1993, Denmark granted regulatory approval for gadodiamide, a non- ionic linear chelate, as an

C. L. Bennett · B. Witherspoon · K. R. Carson · H. S. Thomsen (✉)
SONAR (Southern Network on Adverse Reactions) Program, University of South Carolina
College of Pharmacy, Columbia, SC 29208, USA
e-mail: Henrik.thomsen@regionh.dk

C. L. Bennett
e-mail: bennettc@cop.sc.edu

K. R. Carson
e-mail: Kenneth_R_Carson@rush.edu

imaging agent at a dose of a 0.1 mmol/kg dose for Magnetic Resonance Imaging (MRI) of the central nervous system and the spine and triple doses for brain metastasis evaluations [4]. The approval included warnings against administering to gadodiamide to persons with renal insufficiency. In 1996, Danish Medicines Agency regulatory approval was granted for gadodiamide at a dose of 0.3 mmol/kg for general MR examinations, including angiography [4]. In 1998, the renal insufficiency contra-indication was removed, based on one study reporting no nephrotoxicity among 49 patients with renal insufficiency who had received gadodiamide 0.1 mmol/kg [4]. Subsequently, gadodiamide became the most common GBCA administered in Denmark. Peak gadodiamide use as part of MR examinations occurred between 2002 and 2005 [4].

Prior to March 2006, routine practice at Herlev Hospital in Copenhagen was to perform MR examinations on CKD patients being considered for renal transplantation using gadodiamide. The goal was to visualize the vascular anatomy with gadodiamide doses of 0.3 mmol/kg, standard dose for peripheral run-offs with the MR scanners that were available in the beginning of the decade.

In-person interviews with officials from the Danish Health Ministry, the Patient Insurance Association, the DMA, Danish clinicians, and the son of the index NSF case in Denmark facilitated our understanding about the events that led to the identification and eradication of NSF in Denmark (Table 6.2).

In 2002, a Herlev Hospital nephrologist reported to the Danish Medicines Agency that a 48 year old man had developed severe muscle pain and oliguria immediately following a gadodiamide-enhanced MR angiogram- requiring conversion from peritoneal dialysis to hemodialysis. One month later, a rheumatologist and a dermatologist from Copenhagen reported to the Danish Medicines Agency that a 55 year old CKD female had developed skin, joint, and muscle pains and oliguria immediately following another gadodiamide-enhanced MR angiogram, also necessitating conversion from peritoneal dialysis to hemodialysis. A skin biopsy was read as consistent with an allergic reaction. The patient became wheel-chair bound and died of pulmonary embolism. The Danish Patient Insurance Agency ruled that the disability and subsequent death resulted from gadodiamide exposure and allocated some funds to the family.

In 2003, a radiology resident at Herlev Hospital reviewed records for 104 CKD patients who had undergone gadodiamide-enhanced MR investigations (usually 0.3 mmol/kg) in 2002 and 2003, identifying two patients with nephrotoxicity who had developed muscle pain within days after undergoing the procedure. The report was published in 2005 [5]. The primary purpose of the review was to report on the diagnostic findings, and therefore the clinical follow-up was purposely brief. These were the same two patients who had been reported to the DMA in 2002 [4] The conclusion was that administration of one particular GBCA, gadodiamide, to CKD patients was probably non-toxic and that underlying disease accounted for the findings for the two patients. In 2005, a nephrology resident at Herlev Hospital suspected that an unknown exposure accounted for skin, muscle, and joint abnormalities developing among 10 CKD patients. A dataset was sent to the Regional Health Inspector in Denmark, but no etiologic cause was implicated. Subsequently,

Table 6.1 Gadolinium containing agents and Commercial names (adapted from European Medicines Agency [23])

Generic name	Brand name	Acronym	Chemical structure	Charge	Risk for NSF[c]	Date of FDA/EMA/DMA approval
Gadodiamide	Omniscan[a]	Gd-DTPA-BMA	Linear	Non-ionic	High	FDA approved: 01/1993 (287 mg/ml); DMA Approved: 01/1994
Gadoversetamide	OptiMARK[a]	Gd-DTPA-BMEA	Linear	Non-ionic	High	FDA approved: 12/1999 EMA approved 07/2007
Gadopentetate dimeglumine	Magnevist[a]	Gd-DTPA	Linear	Ionic	High	FDA approved: 06/1988 and 03/2000 DMA approved: 08/1989
Gadobenate dimeglumine	MultiHance[a]	Gd-BOPTA	Linear	Ionic	Medium	FDA approved: 11/2004 DMA approved: 10/1998
Gadoxetic acid disodium salt	Primovist[b] Eovist[a]	Gd-EOB-DTPA	Linear	Ionic	Medium	FDA approved: 07/2008 Not approved in Denmark
Gadofosveset trisodium	Vasovist[b]	Gd-DTPA	Linear	Ionic	Medium	EMA approved: 10/2005 FDA Approved: 12/2008
Gadoteridol	ProHance[a]	Gd-HP-DO3A	Cyclic	Non-ionic	Low	FDA approved: 11/1992 DMA approved: 02/1994
Gadobutrol	Gadovist[b]	Gd-BT-DO3A	Cyclic	Non-ionic	Low	EMA approved: 06/2000 DMA approved: 09/2000 Not FDA approved
Gadoterate meglumine	Dotarem[b]	Gd-DOTA	Cyclic	Ionic	Low	Available in France: 07/1989 DMA approved: 03/1996

[a] Approved by the FDA for use with magnetic resonance imaging in the United States
[b] Approved by the European Medicines Agency for use with enhanced MRI
[c] Risk of NSF as noted by the European Medicines Agency (2007)
(Only Vasovist and Optimark have received multi-country registration in Europe. The other GBCAs approved in Denmark were registered by the Danish Medicines Agency (DMA)) Vasovist is no longer sold in Europe, whereas it is sold under the brandname Ablavar in the US

Table 6.2 Opportunities to recognize the association of gadodiamide administration with NSF development in Denmark (2002–2006)

Event	Action	Initial response	Later action
2002			
Index case develops acute skin toxicity immediately after undergoing a gadodiamide-enhanced MR at Herlev Hospital	Case reported to Danish Medicines Agency	Patient's findings are categorized by the manufacturer as being consistent with underlying disease	Manufacturers are no longer asked to adjudicate adverse event report descriptions
Second NSF case undergoes skin biopsy	Pathologist reviews the biopsy	Pathologist reads the biopsy as being consistent with foreign body reaction	Re-read of the biopsy in 2006 confirms the diagnosis of NSF
Second NSF case	Case reported to the manufacturer of gadodiamide by a dermatologist and a rheumatologist	Manufacturer classifies the case as exacerbation of underlying auto-immune disease	Biopsy reviewed by Shawn Cowper and confirms NSF diagnosis
Index case from Herlev Hospital develops muscle pain immediately after undergoing a gadodiamide-enhanced MR procedure	Case reported to the manufacturer	Manufacturer classifies the case as exacerbation of underlying disease	Skin biopsy was re-read as NSF and gadolinium was identified by scanning electron microscopy
2003			
Second Danish NSF case dies and Danish Patient Insurance Association (PIA) awards large financial compensation	Danish PIA sends report of financial compensation to the manufacturer- and states that patient's death was probably a result of the gadodiamide administration	Manufacturer classifies the death as a consequence of underlying immunologic disease	Patient diagnosed with NSF after death—in 2006
Manufacturer updates Periodic Safety Update Report (PSUR)	The PSUR does not list the first two NSF patients' deaths as serious adverse drug reactions	The PSUR listing could have included the 2002 and 2003 cases as potential fatal adverse drug reactions	Patient's deaths reclassified as a serious adverse drug reaction in 2006
2004			
Similar clinical findings for a CKD patient undergoing a	Radiologist in Texas telephones manufacturer to query	Manufacturer does not link this case with the two index	FDA requests in 2006 that the manufacturer review this case for

(continued)

Table 6.2 (continued)

Event	Action	Initial response	Later action
gadodiamide-enhanced MR procedure in Texas	whether any similar cases have been reported	cases from Herlev Hospital in 2002	possibility of NSF diagnosis
Manufacturer sends a Periodic Safety Update Report to Danish regulatory authorities	All serious adverse drug reactions identified by the manufacturer are described	Details of the two Danish patients and the one Texas patient are not included in this 2004 PSUR prior to 2006	The three patients are reclassified in 2006 as having had biopsy confirmed NSF and are added to a 2006 PSUR
2005			
A radiology resident in radiology published a Herlev Hospital look-back study of 104 CKD patients who underwent gadodiamide-enhanced MR procedures in 2002 and 2003(5)	Medical records and angiograms are reviewed by radiologists at Herlev Hospital	Records of only two patients identify skin and muscle changes following the MR procedure. The records were reviewed for evidence of nephrotoxicity and changes in vascular findings within days of the procedure. Nephrologists attribute the changes to exogenous iron administration	After examining most of these patients in late 2006, the diagnosis of NSF is biopsy confirmed in 8 patients who had gadodiamide administered between 2001 and 2003
A nephrology resident suspects that gadolinium might be the cause of acute skin changes and neuropathic symptoms of peritoneal dialsysis patient exposed to gadodiamide in autumn 2005	Skin biopsy sent to a pathologist for examination for gadolinium in 2005	Methodology to identify Gadolinium in skin biopsy is unavailable in 2005	Scanning electron microscopy identifies gadolinium in biopsy in 2007
Nephrologist suspects that common exposure might account for skin, muscle, and joint changes in 10 CKD patients at Herlev Hospital	Medical record review is done. Summary table created in 2005 includes clinical findings and potential exposures	Gadolinium is listed as an exposure on only two of the 10 case summaries in the 2005 summary table	2006 re-review of the medical records identifies gadodiamide-exposure on all 10 patients

(continued)

Table 6.2 (continued)

Event	Action	Initial response	Later action
A fourth CKD patient develops acute toxicity following the gadodiamide-enhanced MR procedure	Clinicians in Germany report the details of this patient to the gadodiamide manufacturer of acute toxicity following the gadodiamide-enhanced MR procedure	Clinical details are not linked by safety personnel at the manufacturer with the prior three reports	2006- re-review classifies this patient as having had NSF
2006			
A Herlev Hospital nephrologist identifies 20 CKD patients with clinical diagnoses of NSF—all had undergone a gadodiamide— enhanced MR imaging procedure (early March 2006)	The Hospital nephrologist telephones the Danish Medicines Agency and describes the 20 CKD patients as having clinical diagnoses of NSF- all had undergone a gadodiamide-enhanced MR imaging procedure (early March 2006). These reports form the basis for the Danish Medicines Agency dissemination of a statement of concern and are forwarded to the EMA, FDA, and to gadodiamide's manufacturer	All 20 patients were later described in a written communication by the nephrologists to the DMA as clinically suspected NSF cases (Late March 2006). These reports form the basis for the Danish Medicines Agency dissemination of a statement of concern and are forwarded to the EMA, FDA, and to gadodiamide's manufacturer. (May 2006)	Skin biopsies confirm the NSF diagnosis in 13 of these patients. Findings are published as a rapid communication in August in the Journal of the American Society of Nephrology [7] in 2006

in 2006, all of these patients were found to have undergone gadodiamide-enhanced MR procedures and to have biopsy-confirmed NSF diagnoses). Another nephrology resident requested that a dermatopathologist look for gadolinium in a skin biopsy obtained from a patient presenting with skin, joint, and muscle abnormalities after a gadodiamide-enhanced MR angiogram. However, the diagnostic methodology was unavailable at that time.

In January 2006, a Austrian nephrologist described an association between five cases of NSF and prior use of a GBCA. This manuscript described CKD patients in Austria who had developed probable NSF following MR investigations reportedly with gadopeentate dimeglumine, one specific linear chelated GBCA. A subsequently published erratum implicated gadodiamide as the GBCA [6]. In March 2006, the Herlev Hospital nephrologist became the first clinician to report to a national regulatory agency (the Danish Medicines Agency in this instance) information on NSF occurring in CKD patients. The telephone report described 20 CKD patients who had undergone gadodiamide MR investigations at Herlev Hospital, and subsequently had developed what appeared to be NSF. Median time from gadodiamide exposure to NSF was 25 days [7]. A minimum 3.5% NSF risk estimate among gadodiamide-exposed CKD patients was reported. Subsequently, Herlev Hospital discontinued gadodiamide administration to all patients independent of renal function.

In August 2006, clinicians at another Danish hospital, Skejby Hospital, reported that they had not diagnosed any NSF cases, despite routinely imaging CKD patients who were transplant candidates with gadodiamide-enhanced MR angiograms (usually at a dose of 0.1 mmol/kg), although a minority of MR angiograms were enhanced with two other GBCAs.

In October 2006, clinicians from Herlev and Skejby Hospitals in Denmark, manufacturers' representatives for two linear-chelated GBCAs (gadodiamide and gadopentetate dimeglumine), and Danish Medicinees Agency DMA representatives attended a Skejby Hospital workshop. Nephrologists from Skejby Hospital reported that conditions unique to Herlev Hospital had probably resulted in NSF, since similar cases were not recognized at other Danish hospitals. Nonetheless, Skejby Hospital discontinued administering gadodiamide, the GBCA that had been implicated at Herlev Hospital.

A December 2007 review of medical records at Herlev Hospital, augmented by patient interviews, physical examination, and skin biopsies, identified 30 CKD patients with biopsy-confirmed NSF [8–11].

In February 2008, a nephrologist, radiologist, and dermatologist from Herlev Hospital published findings from a retrospective review of 190 CKD patients at their hospital who had received gadodiamide-enhanced MR studies. That study noted a 18% NSF rate (18 of 102 stage 5 CKD patients who had received gadodiamide-enhanced MR examinations) with a mean follow-up of 29 months (range, 16 to 43 months) versus a 0% NSF rate among patients with stages 1 to 4 CKD [9].

In May 2006, the Danish Medicines Agency and employees of gadodiamide's manufacturer reviewed the findings for the NSF patients at Herlev Hospital.(7).. The Danish Medicines Agency had issued a statement indicating potential NSF safety signals had been associated with gadodiamide exposure, although causality was uncertain [4]. This information was communicated to the European Pharmacovigilance Working Party and published on the Danish Medicines Abency's web-site.

In September 2006, the Danish Medicines Agency met with representatives of gadodiamide's manufacturer, who had received 48 NSF case reports worldwide. A case–control study of 38 stage 5 CKD patients had reported mean cumulative lifetime doses of 0.44 mmol/kg in cases versus 0.34 mmol/kg in controls. Among cases, those with severe versus less severe disease had received greater mean cumulative lifetime gadodiamide doses (0.57 versus 0.33 mmol/kg) [10]. The manufacturer again asserted that a causal relationship could not be ascertained.

In February 2008, the Danish Secretary of State for Health and Prevention commissioned the Danish Medicines Agency to review the occurrences of gadodiamide-associated NSF at Herlev Hospital. In March 2008, the DMA's gadodiamide's report was released [11]. The authors reviewed manufacturer's and Danish Medicines Agency actions and concluded that the first NSF safety signals in Denmark had been reported in March 2006, by Peter Marckmann, a nephrologist at Herlev Hospital. The report notes that as of February 29, 2008 the Danish Medicines Agency had received 36 reports with the side effects diagnosis NSF-35 implicated gadodiamide. In 2006, 28 reports had been received-27 of which were from Herlev Hospital and one from Holstebro Hospital in Denmark. One of the reports from Herlev Hospital had already been sent once before, in 2002, but at that time the side effect diagnosis was not indicated as NSF, but had been recorded as muscle pains. In 2007, 7 NSF reports had been received by the Danish Medicines Agency, of which 5 from Herlev Hospital, 1 from Hillerød Hospital and 1 from an unreported hosptial. In 2008, 1 NSF case was reported from Herlev Hospital.

In April 2008, the Health Committee of the Danish Parliament requested that the Danish Health Minister review all regulatory approvals for gadodiamide and pharmacovigilance efforts by the Danish Medicines Agency. The result of this review has not been published.

In November 2008, the Danish Medicines Agency asked the European Committee for Medicinal Products for Human Use (CHMP) to conduct an assessment of the risk of NSF for the non-centrally authorized GBCAs, and to recommend measures that could be taken to reduce NSF risk.

In January 2009, clinicians at Skejby Hospital reported 30 CKD patients with possible NSF. This was based on a comprehensive re-evaluation of their CKD patients. In 2006, these clinicians had reported no CKD patients with NSF. The patients had undergone gadodiamide-enhanced MRIs (dose 0.1 to 0.2 mmol/kg) between 2002 and 2006. Fifteen had died, and skin biopsy confirmed NSF in ten. Clinicians at Odense Hospital in Denmak reported that 16 CKD patients had been exposed to linear chelated GBCAs (either gadodiamide or gadopentetate dimeglumine). Two were diagnosed with NSF-both had received gadodiamide >0.2 mmol/kg. Clinicians at Hillerød and Holstebro Sygehus Hospitals in Denmark reported one gadodiamide-associated and one gadopentetate dimeglumine-associated NSF patient, respectively. Overall, 67 Danish CKD patients had developed probable NSF, of which 43 were biopsy confirmed. All but one had received one or more doses of gadodiamide.

The 2008 Danish Medicines Agency report on NSF had concluded that the first safety signals that had been received by the Agency regarding NSF had occurred in March 2006 when Marckmann, the nephrology resident, had reported 20 NSF cases to the Danish Medicines Agency.

In spring 2009, the Danish Minister of Health requested that an independent investigation be performed by an attorney regarding handling of the gadodiamide/NSF cases by the Danish Medicines Agency, the Danish Ministry of

Health and the Danish National Health authorities. The report was completed in November 2010 and found delays in reporting of safety concerns by the Agency, the Ministry, and the Health Authorities.

6.1.1 European Actions

In February 2007, the European Adverse Drug Reaction Council, the Danish Medicines Agency, and gadodiamide's manufacturer warned that gadodiamide was contra-indicated among patients with severe renal disease, while for other GBCAs, caution in this setting was advised. At that time, NSF had only been reported after exposure to two GBCAs, gadovertisamide and gadodiamide.

In June 2007, the Council advised against use of another GBCA, gadopentetate dimeglumine among severe CKD patients and requested manufacturers of other GBCAs indicate why similar contra-indications should not be mandated. However, the manufacturers of the other GBCAs rejected that request, stating that NSF risks were observed when GBCAs were administered at greater than regulatory approved dosages.

In December 2007, the European Medicines Acency's Scientific Advice Group for Diagnostics classified three GBCAs (gadopentetate dimeglumine, gadoversetamide, and gadodiamide) as high risk- all three were linear-chelated agents and the last two non-ionic. Medium-risk agents included gadofosveset trisodium, gadoxetic acid disodium salt, and gadobenate dimeglumine—all three were linear-chelated and ionic agents. Low-risk agents were gadoterate meglumine, gadoteridol, and gadobutrol- all three were cyclic chelated and the last two were non-ionic.

In November 2009, the European Medicines Agency completed a review on NSF and GBCAs. The Committee on Human Medicines Products (CHMP) agreed with the Scientific Advice Group classification of gadolinium-containing contrast agents into high-, medium- and low-risk agents based on their risk of causing NSF. However, the CHMP recognised that within the high-risk group, the risk of NSF with gadoversetamide and gadodiamide appeared higher than with gadopentetic acid, based on physicochemical properties, studies in animals and the number of cases of NSF reported worldwide. The Committee concluded that an additional factor that may contribute to the risk of NSF is the way these medicines are used (such as dose, duration of administration, and administration with multiple scans). The Committee recommended contraindications in patients with severe kidney problems, in patients who are scheduled for or have recently received a liver transplant and in newborn babies up to four weeks of age. To minimize the risk of using high-risk GBCA agents in patients with unknown kidney problems, the CHMP advised that patients should always be screened for kidney problems using laboratory tests before use. The CHMP also recommended that women should discontinue breastfeeding for at least 24 hours after a scan.

Finally, the CHMP recommended that the prescribing information of all gadolinium-containing contrast agents should include a warning that the elderly may be at particular risk of NSF due to impaired ability of their kidneys to clear gadolinium from the body; a statement that there is no evidence to support the initiation of haemodialysis to prevent or treat NSF in patients not already undergoing haemodialysis; and a statement that the type and dose of contrast agent used should be recorded. This opinion was subsequently approved by the European Medicines Agency.

6.1.2 Actions of the Manufacturer of Gadodiamide

On May 9th 2006, the manufacturer of gadodiamide forwarded a safety alert from the manufacturer of gadodiamide to national health authorities worldwide, including the Danish Medicines Agency. This alert identified an association between gadodiamide administration and NSF development among CKD stage 5 patients, although a causal relationship could not be confirmed.

In February 2008, the Danish Medicines Agency requested that gadodiamide's manufacturer comment upon Danish press allegations that safety information from gadodiamide's manufacturer had been withheld from Danish radiologists. In March 2008, the manufacturer stated that in their opinion in vitro and in vivo assessments did not support conclusions that safety concerns were greater with gadodiamide versus other GBCAs and that reporting of large numbers of gadodiamide-associated NSF cases was biased by incomplete reporting and confounding with effects of other GBCAs.

In 2009, the manufacturer of gadodiamide initiated a libel lawsuit against Henrik Thomsen, the senior radiologist at Herlev Hospital who had been first author or senior author on the majority of publications on gadodiamimde administration to CKD patients at Herlev Hospital since 1999. Thomsen stated that the lawsuit represented an attempt to "stifle" him from reporting on the activities of the manufacturer with respect to gadodiamide and subsequent NSF development.

In February 2010, this lawsuit, which cost the manufacturer at least $1 million, was settled, with the manufacturer paying the court costs of Dr. Thomsen.Before the settlement, Thomsen had indicated that he would countersue the manufacturer for defamation of character.

6.2 Basic Science Considerations

Scanning electron microscopy with energy dispersive spectroscopy identified gadolinium in skin biopsies from NSF patients at Herlev Hospital in 2006 [12, 13]. Inductively coupled plasma mass spectrometry, with improved sensitivity and gravimetric methodology, later confirmed significant gadolinium accumulation within the tissues of NSF patients [14, 15]. Metal ions compete with gadolinium for ligand binding, a phenomenon called transmetallation. It is believed this event probably occurs more readily with non-ionic linear chelates that have lesser thermodynamic and kinetic stabilities. Impaired renal function and higher temperatures enhance transmetallation, by increasing GBCA's half-life from 1.5 to 30 h [16–18]. Shifts in iron stores following exposure to some GBCAs might involve transmetallation [19]. Rodent models and human studies demonstrate higher levels of residual gadolinium with linear versus cyclic gadolinium chelates after GBCA injection [20].

6.3 Explanations for the Danish Findings

Product and clinician-specific factors may account for the high prevalence and the high caseload of gadodiamide-associated NSF at Herlev Hospital. During 2002–2006, Herlev Hospital accounted for the most gadodiamide use in Denmark. Beginning in November 2001 at Herlev Hospital (when a MR scanner was first installed there), gadodiamide was administered to kidney transplant candidates (a unique practice internationally) in an effort to identify compromised vascular systems. Following a 2006 change from gadodiamide to macrocyclic GBCAs, no new NSF cases at Herlev Hospital were reported. Of note, for 15 CKD stage 5 patients in whom high resolution of the vasculature was clinically indicated, high-dose MR angiograms with macrocyclic GBCAs were performed at Herlev Hospital after 2006- with no NSF instances.

Prior to 2009, officials in Denmark concluded that conditions at Herlev Hospital (administration of gadodiamide at doses of 0.3 mmol/kg to CKD patients who were candidates for renal transplantation) accounted for the observation that all NSF cases in Denmark were from Herlev Hospital. In 2009, a look-back study conducted by clinicians at Skejby Hospital in Copenhagen concluded otherwise. This study identified 10 biopsy-confirmed CKD patients from Skejby Hospital who had developed NSF between 2002 and 2006. All had undergone gadodiamide-enhanced MR angiograms (dose of 0.1 to 0.2 mmol/kg). An additional 20 CKD patients with potential gadodiamide-associated NSF at Skejby Hospital were identified, although skin biopsies had not been performed. This finding provided support for the observation that NSF was a complication that any CKD patient can develop- rather than being unique to patients at Herlev Hospital. Forty CKD patients have been reported from Danish hospitals other than Herlev. The Danish Parliament had established a national compensation fund for all Danish persons who developed in NSF in Denmark.

6.4 International Considerations

In 2003, 2004, and 2005 when the manufacturer of gadodiamide received adverse event reports of similar cases from Herlev Hospital, Texas, and Germany, the manufacturer's assessment was that each case was unlikely to have been caused by gadodiamide. Subsequently, biopsy-confirmed NSF was diagnosed in these patients. Between 2003 and 2006, reports of 40 persons with CKD, hepatorenal syndrome internationally with renal insufficiency, or acute kidney injury postulated causative factors for NSF as contaminated dialysate or elaborated toxins; [17, 18] antiphospholipid antibodies [16]; volume overload [16]; side-effects of cyclosporine, erythropoietin, or angiotensin converting enzyme inhibitors;(12, 13) or infectious agents [14].

The time-line in Denmark of NSF cases is similar to timelines reported by the FDA and GBCA manufacturers (Fig. 6.1A, B). However, additional NSF cases were reported based on registry findings from settings other than Herlev Hospital after March 2006. NSF cases at other hospitals were associated with other GBCAs, primarily the linear-chelated GBCA gadopentate dimeglumine; and the prevalence of GBCA-associated NSF among stage 5 CKD patients at other hospitals internationally range from 3 to 5%, based on registry studies, versus 18% at Herlev Hospital, based on a systematic review of all patient records and patient examinations. The difference in epidemiologic rate estimates results in large part from the methodologic differences. Herlev Hospital conducted formal evaluations of all CKD patients who underwent GBCA-enhanced MR examinations between 2001 and 2007, while the other hospitals in Denmark primarily relied on registry data.

The Danish Medicines Agency, in collaboration with the Food and Drug Administration in the United States, and the European Medicines Agency served an international leadership role in identifying NSF and in leading the responses of other regulatory agencies. The May 2006 Internet-disseminated safety notification from the Danish Medicines Agency was coordinated with notifications from the European Medicines Agency and the Food and Drug Administration in June 2006 [11, 21, 22]. In 2007, the Danish Medicines A and EMA, in response to recommendations from the European Medicine's Agency Scientific Advisory Group for Diagnostics, designated three linear GBCAs as high NSF risk among CKD stage 4–5 patients. Regulatory notifications from Denmark were mirrored by the European Medicines Agency, but not the Food and Drug Administration, warning against administering three GBCAs [23] (gadodiamide, gadopentetate dimeglumine, and gadoversetamide) to CKD stage 4–5 patients and that medium-risk GBCAs include ionic linear chelates (gadobenate dimeglumine, gadoexetic acid disodium salt and gadofosveset trisodium); and that low-risk GBCAs include macrocyclic chelates. An initial Food and Drug Administraion Advisory in 2007 warns of NSF risk following administration of any GBCA to patients with CKD stage 4–5, acute kidney injury including hepato-renal syndrome, or post-liver transplantation [3].

6.5 Summary

The international medical community benefited tremendously from important pharmacovigilance performed at Herlev Hospital in Copenhagen and safety actions by the European Medicines Agency taken in response to Danish Medicines Agency notifications. Few new cases of NSF developed year among CKD patients as a

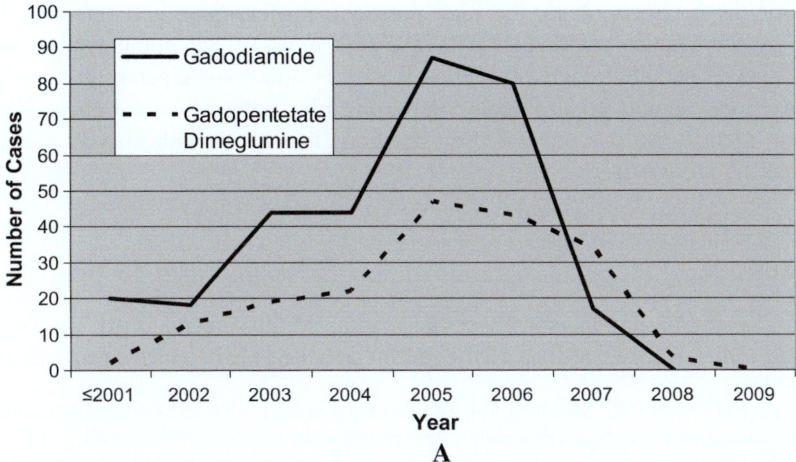

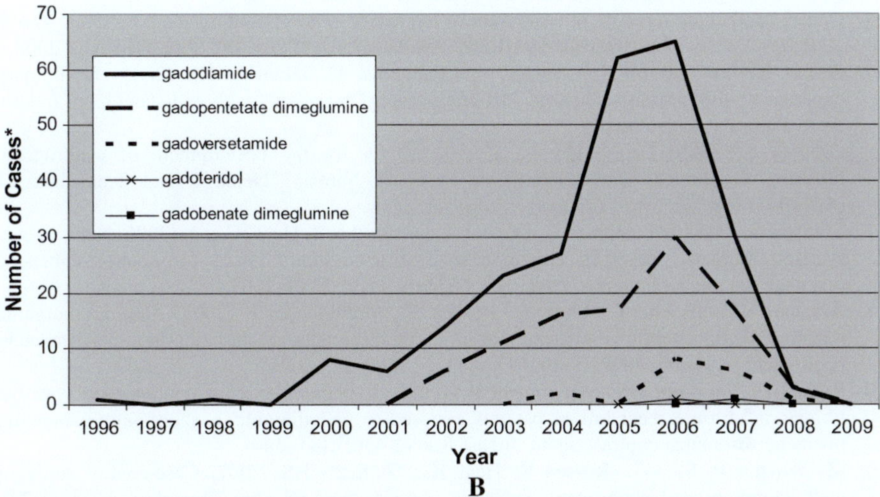

Fig. 6.1 **A** Number of cases by year in the manufacturer's database for gadodiamide and gadopentetate dimeglumine. (Data provided by the manufacturer's of gadodiamide and gadopentetate dimeglumine). **B** Number of cases* of GBCA-associated NSF each year by product as identified in the Food and Drug Administration's Medwatch database. *Only cases with a confirmed event date included in the figure. FDA have received a total of 1209 reports. (Data taken from the FDA's MedWatch Adverse Event Reporting System)

result of these efforts. Also, the high personal, professional, and financial costs faced by the Danish radiologist who oversaw most of the initial reports of an association of gadodiamide with NSF at Herlev Hospital are apparent in retrospect. Future efforts should go further in supporting clinicians who take huge risks to publicly identify serious adverse drug reactions that occur with heavily marketed pharmaceutical agents.

References

1. Lasser KE, Allen PD, Woolhandler SJ, Himmelstein DU, Wolfe SM, Bor DH (2002) Timing of new black box warnings and withdrawals for prescription medications. JAMA 287:2215–2220
2. Cowper SE, Robin HS, Steinberg SM, Su LD, Gupta S, LeBoit PE (2000) Scleromyxoedema-like cutaneous diseases in renal-dialysis patients. Lancet 356(9234):1000–1001
3. FDA. Information on Gadolinium-Containing Contrast Agents. 2007 May;http://www.fda.gov/cder/drug/infopage/gcca/default.htm Accessed April 8, 2008.
4. Danish Medicines Agency. Investigation of the safety of MRI contrast medium Omniscan®. 2006;http://www.dkma.dk/1024/visUKLSArtikel.asp?artikelID=8931. Accessed Sept 2008
5. Perriss R, Lokkegaard H, Logager V, Chabanova E, Thomsen HS (2005) Preliminary experience with contrast-enhanced MR angiography in patients with end-stage renal failure. Acad Radiol 12(5):652–657
6. Grobner T (2006) Gadolinium—a specific trigger for the development of nephrogenic fibrosing dermopathy and nephrogenic systemic fibrosis? Nephrol Dial Transplant 21(4):1104–1108
7. Marckmann P, Skov L, Rossen K, Dupont A, Damholt MB, Heaf JG et al (2006) Nephrogenic systemic fibrosis: suspected causative role of gadodiamide used for contrast-enhanced magnetic resonance imaging. J Am Soc Nephrol 17(9):2359–2362
8. Abraham JL, Thakral C, Skov L, Rossen K, Marckmann P (2008) Dermal inorganic gadolinium concentrations: evidence for in vivo transmetallation and long-term persistence in nephrogenic systemic fibrosis. Br J Dermatol 158(2):273–280
9. Rydahl C, Thomsen HS, Marckmann P (2008) High prevalence of nephrogenic systemic fibrosis in chronic renal failure patients exposed to gadodiamide, a gadolinium-containing magnetic resonance contrast agent. Invest Radiol 43(2):141–144
10. Marckmann P, Skov L, Rossen K, Heaf JG, Thomsen HS (2007) Case-control study of gadodiamide-related nephrogenic systemic fibrosis. Nephrol Dial Transplant 22(11):3174–3178
11. The Danish Medicine Agency Report on the contrast agent Omniscan®. 2008 March 27.
12. Boyd AS, Zic JA, Abraham JL (2007) Gadolinium deposition in nephrogenic fibrosing dermopathy. J Am Acad Dermatol 56(1):27–30
13. High WA, Ayers RA, Chandler J, Zito G, Cowper SE (2007) Gadolinium is detectable within the tissue of patients with nephrogenic systemic fibrosis. J Am Acad Dermatol 56(1):21–26
14. High WA, Ayers RA, Cowper SE (2007) Gadolinium is quantifiable within the tissue of patients with nephrogenic systemic fibrosis. J Am Acad Dermatol 56(4):710–712
15. Khurana A Jr, JFG, High WA, (2008) Quantification of gadolinium in nephrogenic systemic fibrosis: re-examination of a reported cohort with analysis of clinical factors. J Am Acad Dermatol 59(2):218–224
16. Joffe P, Thomsen HS, Meusel M (1998) Pharmacokinetics of gadodiamide injection in patients with severe renal insufficiency and patients undergoing hemodialysis or continuous ambulatory peritoneal dialysis. Acad Radiol 5:491–502

17. Tombach B, Bremer C, Reimer P, Schaefer RM, Ebert W, Geens V et al (2000) Pharmacokinetics of 1 m gadobutrol in patients with chronic renal failure. Invest Radiol 35:35–40
18. Townsend RR, Cohen DL, Katholi R, Swan SK, Davies BE, Bensel K et al (2000) Safety of intravenous gadolinium (Gd-BOPTA) infusion in patients with renal insufficiency. Am J Kidney Dis 36:1207–1212
19. Swaminathan S, Horn TD, Pellowski D, Abul-Ezz S, Bornhorst JA, Viswamitra S, et al (2007) Nephrogenic systemic fibrosis, gadolinium, and iron mobilization. N Engl J Med Aug 16;357(7):720–722
20. Sieber MA, Pietsch H, Walter J, Haider W, Frenzel T, Weinmann HJ (2008) A preclinical study to investigate the development of nephrogenic systemic fibrosis: a possible role for gadolinium-based contrast media. Invest Radiol 43(1):65–75
21. FDA. Public Health Advisory. Gadolinium-containing Contrast Agency for Magnetic Resonance Imaging (MRI): Omniscan, OptiMARK, Magnevist, ProHance and MultiHance. 2006. http://www.contrastdye-lawsuit.com/pdfs/FDA.PHA.June.2006.pdf. Accessed 1 Aug 2009
22. EMEA. Gadolinium-containing MRI contrast agents and Nephrogenic Systemic Fibrosis (NSF). 2007. http://www.ismrm.org/special/EMEA1.pdf. Accessed 28 Sep 2008
23. The Medicines and Healthcare products Regulatory Agency website. Nephrogenic systemic fibrosis (NSF) and gadolinium-containing MRI contrast agents. 2007. http://www.mhra.gov.uk/home/groups/pl-p/documents/websiteresources/con2030231.pdf. Accessed 30 Dec 2007

Charles L. Bennett MD, Ph.D., MPP, SmartState Chair and Frank P. and Josie M. Fletcher Chair of Medication Safety and Efficacy and Director, SmartState Center for Medication Safety and Efficacy, is also a Visiting Scholar at the City of Hope National Cancer Institute Designated Comprehensive Cancer Center in Duarte, California and is the co-editor of this book, Cancer Policy (2nd Edition). Dr. Bennett is a Phi Beta Kappa and High Honors graduate in mathematics from Swarthmore College, earned his medical degree in 1981 from the University of Pennsylvania Perelman School of Medicine, and completed internal medicine, hematology, and oncology training at the Michael Reese Hospital and the University of Chicago Pritzger School of Medicine before completing his Ph.D. and Masters In Public Policy degrees with honors in social science at the RAND Pardee Graduate School of Public Policy in Santa Monica, California. He has led a 20-year National Institutes of Health funded pharmacovigilance called the Research on Adverse Drug events And Reports (RADAR) and subsequently called to Southern Network on Adverse drug Reactions (SONAR) at the University of South Carolina College of Pharmacy.

Bartlett Witherspoon MBA is a third-year medical student at the Medical University of South Carolina and a graduate of Vanderbilt University's Master's in Business Administration program. He is an active co-investigator with Dr. Bennett and the SONAR project and has been a lead co-investigator on published manuscripts on fluoroquinolone-associated disability and on biosimilar oncology products.

Kenneth R. Carson MD, Ph.D. is Assistant Professor of Medicine at the Rush University School of Medicine and is also Vice-President for Tempus, Incorporated. He is a hematologist/oncologist trained at Northwestern University with a Ph.D. in public health from the University of Illinois at Chicago. He is a long-time collaborator with RADAR and SONAR and was the first author on the important 2009 manuscript in Blood describing 57 cases of rituximab-associated progressive multi-focal leukoencephalopathy.

Henrik S. Thomsen MD received his medical education from the University of CHP. He is a board-certified radiologist and served as chair of the radiology department at CPH University Hospital Herlev from 2002 to 2008. He was the director of diagnostic sciences for the faculty of health in 2000. He is the author or co-author of 625 manuscripts including original papers, reviews, and book chapters in topics ranging from uroradiology to musculoskeletal radiology and contrast media. He is a member of the editorial board of 4 international journals and chief editor of Acta Radiologica. He is also the recipient of numerous awards such as the Lifetime Achievement Award for the Society of Uroradiology and the Harry Fischer Award as well as the Torsten Almén Award.

Rituximab-Associated Progressive Multifocal Leukoencephalopathy: A Twenty-Year Update

Charles L. Bennett, Bartlett Witherspoon, and Kenneth R. Carson

7.1 Introduction

Progressive multifocal leukoencephalopathy (PML) is a John-Cunningham virus-related central nervous system that is rarely observed in persons treated with the anti-CD20 monoclonal antibody, rituximab [1-3]. Rituximab-associated PML presents with altered central nervous system function, memory loss, speech defects, and/or confusion—findings commonly associated with Alzheimer's disease. Onset usually occurs within months of rituximab initiation and death usually occurs within weeks. In 2002, 2006, and 2009, two, one, and one case of rituximab-associated PML were reported in the setting of stem cell transplantation and cancer, systemic lupus erythematosus, and rheumatoid arthritis, respectively. In 2009, a case series of 52 persons with lymphoma and 5 patients with rheumatologic or immunologic diseases with rituximab-associated PML was reported. Beginning in 2011, epidemiologic findings for rituximab-associated PML were reported. The United States' and European Marketing Authorization Holders provide Periodic Safety Update Reports on rituximab-associated PML. We review rituximab-associated PML clinical, epidemiologic, and safety findings. Our aim is to provide a comprehensive overview of rituximab-associated PML and to address any ongoing related safety concerns.

C. L. Bennett · B. Witherspoon · K. R. Carson (✉)
SONAR (Southern Network on Adverse Reactions) Program, University of South Carolina College of Pharmacy, Columbia, SC 29208, USA
e-mail: Kenneth_R_Carson@rush.edu

C. L. Bennett
e-mail: bennettc@cop.sc.edu

7.2   Methods

Original data on rituximab-associated PML generated by two National Cancer Institute funded pharmacovigilance programs, the Research on Adverse Drug Events and Reports ((RADAR) 1998–2010) and the Southern Network on Adverse Drug Reactions (SONAR 20101–2020), were reviewed. Additional data on case series and epidemiologic studies were sought via PubMed searches (MeSH terms: PML; hematologic malignancy (general and specific cancer diagnoses) and rheumatologic diseases (MeSH terms: PML; specific rheumatologic diseases) for the years 1996 to 2019. Case reports were excluded as this information was duplicated in the FDA's Adverse Event Reporting System (FAERS) database and Periodic Safety Update Reports produced by Marketing Authorization Holders in Europe and the United States (2006–2019). Pharmacovigilance information and safety-related advisories for rituximab-associated PML were obtained from websites maintained by the Food and Drug Administration and the European Medicines Agency.

7.3   Results

PubMed searches failed to identify any clinical or epidemiologic data that were not duplicated in RADAR or SONAR databases on rituximab-associated PML. We therefore report on primary data contained in a RADAR national dataset and three SONAR VA datasets and reviews of rituximab-associated PML in FAERS and Manufacturer Authorization Holder's PSURs.

7.4   Case Series

RADAR reported a larger case series of 57 HIV-negative patients with confirmed or clinically diagnosed cases of PML. Data were obtained from FAERS, the manufacturer, and physicians (search period from 1997 to 2008). Overall, 52 patients with lymphoproliferative disorders, 2 patients with systemic lupus erythematosus, 1 patient with rheumatoid arthritis, 1 patient with an idiopathic autoimmune pancytopenia, and 1 patient with immune thrombocytopenia developed PML after treatment with rituximab and other agents. Other treatments included hematopoietic stem cell transplantation (7 patients), purine analogs (26 patients), or alkylating agents (39 patients). One patient with an autoimmune hemolytic anemia developed PML after treatment with corticosteroids and rituximab, and 1 patient with an autoimmune pancytopenia developed PML after treatment with corticosteroids, azathioprine, and rituximab. Median time from last rituximab dose to PML diagnosis was 5.5 months. Median time to death after PML diagnosis was 2.0 months. The case-fatality rate was 91%.

Based on review of electronic databases, SONAR identified 23 PML patients among patients who received care for NHL at any Veterans Administration Medical Center between 1998 and 2001. Of these, four were excluded (HIV positive (four), diagnosed with PML prior to NHL (five), and never received rituximab (seven) (Fig. 7.1). All seven PML cases were male and non-Hispanic. (Table 7.1) Among the seven rituximab-treated NHL patients who developed rituximab-associated PML, the median age at the time of NHL diagnosis was 65.3 years, the median age at death was 65.4 years, the median time to PML diagnosis from NHL diagnosis was 43.2 months, the median time to death from PML diagnosis was 2.0 months, and the median time to PML diagnosis from first rituximab dose was 9.7 months. The case-fatality rate was 100%.

SONAR identified nine patients with rheumatoid arthritis and confirmed diagnoses of PML in the FAERS dataset. Eight were women. Their overall mean age was 65 years (range, 50–83 years). All nine patients had a diagnosis of RA for 3 years and all were HIV-negative. Additionally, they all had $\geq$ 1 known risk factor for PML independent of rituximab, including Sjögren syndrome ($n = 4$), malignancy ($n = 2$), prior/concomitant therapy with disease-modifying anti-rheumatic drugs $n = 9$; most commonly methotrexate), and treatment with 2 prior TNF inhibitors ($n = 4$). The case-fatality rate was 67%.

SONAR identified 231 confirmed or clinically diagnosed cases of PML associated with rituximab treatment in HIV-negative patients during 1999 and 2012 in the FAERS dataset. The majority of patients had received rituximab for hematologic malignancies such as NHL (58.8%) and CLL (28.4%). Non-Hodgkin's lymphoma disorders included follicular lymphoma, diffuse large B-cell lymphoma (DLBCL), mantle cell lymphoma, Waldenstrom's macroglobulinemia, and marginal zone lymphoma. PML was confirmed by brain MRI scans identifying lesions

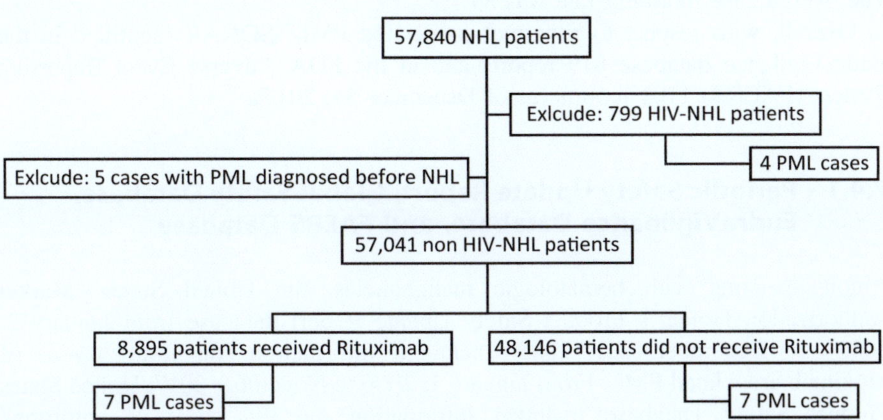

Fig. 7.1 Exclusion diagram of the non-Hodgkin's lymphoma—progressive multifocal leukoencephalopathy cohort (2003–2011). SONAR Pilot Data on Rituximab-associated PML in the setting of hematologic malignancies

Table 7.1 Characteristics of NHL patients in the VA medical system with versus without rituximab treatment (2003–2011)

	PML patients with rituximab ($n = 7$)	PML patients without rituximab ($n = 7$)
Male (%)	7 (100)	7 (100)
Died (%)	6 (85.7)	6 (85.7)
Mean age in years at death (sd)	65.1 years (6.9)	67.3 years (6.6)
Mean age at PML diagnosis (sd)	65.5 years (6.7)	68.7 years (7.3)
Mean time to death from lymphoma diagnosis (sd)	34.0 mo (17.8)	26.6 mo (27.5)
Mean time to death from PML diagnosis (sd)	5.1 mo (8.6)	3.0 (3.9)
Mean time to PML diagnosis from lymphoma diagnosis (sd)	36.2 mo (27.6)	31.0 mo (31.7)
Mean time to PML diagnosis from first rituximab dose (sd)	14.9mo (22.8)	N/A

consistent with PML and positive JC virus CSF PCR (67.5%), brain biopsy (34.6%), or autopsy (7.8%). Twenty-five patients (10.8%) underwent prior transplantation (autologous stem cell transplant, n = 12; allogenic stem cell transplant, n = 8; solid organ transplant, n = 5). Patients were a median age of 64.5 years (range, 19–90 years). Patients received a median of 6 rituximab infusions (range, 1–24 infusions). The median time from first dose of rituximab to diagnosis of PML was 15 months (range, 0.5–128 months) and the median time to diagnosis of PML following the last dose of rituximab was 4 months (range, 0–65 months). The median time from PML diagnosis to death was 2 months (range, 0–14 months). The overall case mortality rate was 89.1%.

Overall, with respect to rituximab-associated PML, SONAR identified in the EudraVigilance database 819 reports and in the FDA Adverse Event Reporting System (FAERS) 1101 reports (as of December 31, 2017).

7.4.1 Periodic Safety Update Report, Global Safety Database, EudraViglinance Database, and FAERS Database

Among persons with hematologic malignancies, the United States' Market Authorization Holder's Product Safety Update Report database from January 1, 2002 to December 31, 2005 included information on four cases of rituximab-associated PML. From January 1, 2006 to November 2017, United States Product Safety Database included information on 338 cases of confirmed rituximab-associated PML cases, including 221 and 117 confirmed cases of PML in patients treated with rituximab for NHL and CLL (chronic lymphocytic leukemia), respectively [4]. Larger numbers of cases of rituximab-associated PML were included in the European Union's Market Authorization Holder Global Safety

Database—734 cases of confirmed and unconfirmed PML, including 144 cases with CLL (111 confirmed) and 356 with PML (215 confirmed) (Roche, data on file). For confirmed cases of rituximab-associated PML associated with rheumatoid arthritis, granulomatosis polyangiitis, and microscopic pokyangiiitis, the European Marketing Authorization Holder's global safety database contained information on 54 cases with rheumatoid arthritis and ten with GPA/MPA). On December 31, 2017, the EudraVigilance database contained 819 reports of PML for rituximab (1998–2017), while the FDA Adverse Event Reporting System (FAERS) database contained 1101 reports (1996–2017).

7.5 Epidemiologic Studies

SONAR conducted a retrospective cohort study using electronic medical records from the Veteran's Health Administration [5]. The study compared a comprehensive cohort of NHL patients who received rituximab and developed PML compared to a cohort of NHL patients who did not receive rituximab and developed PML (2003 to 2011). Patients who were HIV positive and/or who were diagnosed with PML prior to being diagnosed with NHL were excluded. Patients receiving either CHOP-R or maintenance rituximab were grouped into the rituximab arm. SONAR identified 57,840 NHL patients who received care in the national VA medical system. Of these, 799 (1.4%) were HIV positive. Of the remaining 57,041; 8,895 (15.6%) received rituximab and 48,146 (84.4%) did not receive rituximab. The rate of PML cases among NHL patients who received rituximab was 7 per 8,895 NHL patients (7.8 per 10,000) while the rate of PML cases among NHL patients who did not receive rituximab was 7 per 48,146 NHL patients (1.5 per 10,000). This results in a crude Relative Risk (RR) of 5.4 (95% CI: 1.9–15.4).

SONAR conducted a second epidemiologic study of PML in rituximab-treated lymphoma patients diagnosed between 1999 and 2012 at a Veterans Medical Center [6]. Of 61,132 HIV-negative patients with a primary diagnosis of Hodgkin's disease (HD) or NHL, 10,459 patients (17.1%) received rituximab. Of 12 patients (0.02%) who developed PML, 5 were treated with rituximab (8 per 10,000 rtixuximab-treated patients) while 7 received non-rituximab treatment (1.1 per 10,000 rituximab-treated patients). This led to a statistically significant unadjusted relative risk (RR) of 3.5 (95% CI, 1.1–10.9).

SONAR conducted a third epidemiologic study to evaluate the risk of developing PML in rituximab-treated, HIV-negative, Veteran patients diagnosed with CLL [2]. CLL patients ($N = 26,597$) were again identified using electronic medical records from the years 2003 to 2011. PML developed in 4 of 2,425 rituximab-treated patients (16.5 per 10,000) and 2 of 24,172 patients who were not treated with rituximab (0.8 per 10,000; unadjusted RR = 19.9; 95% CI, 3.6–108.8; $p < 0.05$). There was an attributable risk of 15.7 per 10,000 HIV-negative rituximab-treated patients with CLL.

From the first rituximab exposure in RA clinical trials in 2002 up to a cutoff date of 17 November 2015, the Marketing Authorization Holder's global safety database contains information on eleven confirmed PML cases in autoimmune disorders approved for rituximab treatment (nine persons with RA, one with granulomatous polyarthritis (GPA), and one with microscopic polyangiitis (MPA)) [4]. The nine confirmed PML cases in patients with RA correspond to an estimated reported rate of 0.3 cases per 10,000 rituximab-treated RA patients, based on an estimated exposure of 351,396 unique patients treated with rituximab between 2006 (first approval in RA) and 2015, although underreporting rates are estimated at 1–10%. One of nine reported cases was from a manufacturer sponsored RA clinical trial program and occurred five years after the first rituximab dose and 18 months since the last dose, in a patient with a history of malignancy. No PML cases occurred in the double-blind treatment period or control arms of the RA clinical trial program. Eight cases were obtained from spontaneous post-marketing reports submitted to the manufacturer.

7.5.1 PML-Related Safety Notifications from Market Authorization Holders for Rituximab in the US and Europe

In 2009 in the United States, the Marketing Authorization Holder for rituximab and the FDA agreed that Marketing Authorization Holder would report: cumulative summaries of all expedited reports of rituximab-associated PML with results of questionnaires and active attempts to solicit data on such events; results of ongoing analyses to characterize observed rates of PML within all non-HIV-related specific disease categories in which PML has occurred rituximab administration; a comparison of observed rates of PML among those who have and who have not received rituximab to detect trends and estimated rates of PML with evaluation for possible risk factors, e.g., duration of rituximab exposure and results of proposed and ongoing pharmacoepidemiologic evaluations. This Post-Marketing Commitment was due in 2018, but public dissemination of the findings has not yet occurred. The Marketing Authorization Holder also agreed to encourage health care providers to dispense a Medication Guide to each patient who receives rituximab. This Medication Guide is a brief overview of rituximab and, like all Medication Guides, starts with important toxicity information (see Table 7.1) Similarly, in Europe, the marketing authorization holder initiated a Card program requiring all rituximab-treated patients who have a diagnosis of RA, GPA, or MPA to carry a Card with relevant patient information and to give this card to any provider if symptoms of PML arise. No similar safety effort occurs in the setting of hematologic malignancies (Table 7.2).

Table 7.2 Safety notifications for rituximab-associated PML in the US, EU, and Australia

United States

A Medication Guide that is meant to be given to each persons who receives rituximab states: What is the most important information I should know about rituximab? Rituximab can cause serious side effects that can lead to death, including:

Progressive Multifocal Leukoencephalopathy (PML). PML is a rare, serious brain infection caused by a virus that can happen in people who receive rituximab. People with weakened immune systems can get PML. PML can result in death or severe disability. There is no known treatment, prevention, or cure for PML. Tell your healthcare provider right away if you have any new or worsening symptoms or if anyone close to you notices these symptoms: confusion; dizziness or loss of balance; difficulty walking or talking; decreased strength or weakness on one side of your body; or vision problems

Boxed Warning

In 2009, the FDA-approved product label added a Boxed Warning as follows: Progressive Multifocal Leukoencephalopathy (PML): JC virus infection resulting in PML and death has been reported in patients treated with rituximab

Europe

In 2009, the European Medicines Agency required the manufacturer of rituximab to revise the summary of product characteristics (SmPC) to include the following:

The company marketing rituximab will provide doctors and patients who receive rituximab for rheumatoid arthritis, granulomatous polyangiitis, or microscopic polyangiitis or pemphigus with educational material on the risk of infection including of a rare severe infection known as progressive multifocal leukoencephalopathy (PML). These patients are also to receive an alert card, which they are to carry at all times, instructing them to contact their doctor immediately if they experience symptoms of infection. This safety requirement is in place today. It is important to note that neither the summary of product characteristics or the alert card information applies to persons with hematologic malignancies who receive rituximab

7.6 Discussion

These studies are the first to provide detailed clinical and epidemiologic data for rituximab-associated PML. The findings place rituximab-associated PML in context —it is a almost universally fatal ADR that occurs between 5 and 10-times more often among rituximab-treated patients with hematologic malignancies versus patients with hematologic malignancies who do not receive rituximab. In contrast, there are insufficient data to estimate whether PML occurs at an increased rate among rituximab-treated patients with RA, GPA, or MPA.

Our findings have several implications. The various case series show that rituximab-associated PML almost always results in death within weeks to months of onset. As part of FDA mandated post-marketing risk-management efforts, the Marketing Authorization Holder reported that by 2017, 377 rituximab-treated patients with hematologic malignancies had developed PML although updated findings on patient who developed rituximab-associated PML since 2017 have not been reported in the various data sets. Overall, our findings reinforce the importance of conducting epidemiologic studies. Among rituximab-treated persons, the estimate incidence of PML is 15.7, 7.8, and 0.3 per 10,000 persons with non-Hodgkin's lymphoma, CLL, and RA, respectively, although the CLL case numbers are subject to high rates of underreporting in voluntary databases that are managed in Europe and in the United States.

Safety notifications related to rituximab and PML for persons with hematologic malignancies differ in the United States, Europe, and Australia. In the United States, the Marketing Authorization Holder includes Boxed Warnings about rituximab-associated PML among persons with hematologic malignancies as well as among persons with rheumatologic diseases. In contrast, in Europe, the Marketing Authorization Holder reports that rare cases of rituximab-associated PML have been seen among persons with rheumatologic diseases, but an association with hematologic malignancies is not noted in the product label. International harmonization of rituximab-associated PML safety warnings should be considered. In this instance, the United States warnings should be revised to parallel the safety warnings of Europe for this toxicity. This harmonization should be extended to include all regulatory approved rituximab biosimilars, several of which are being marketed in these three regions for varying clinical indications. Specifically, it is time for the Boxed Warning for rituximab-associated PML to be moved to the Warnings and Precautions section in the United States—mirroring the safety language that is disseminated in Europe. Boxed Warnings for possibly or even probably unrelated clinical events are more harmful than helpful to patients who receive rituximab.

References

1. Bennett CL (2011) Pharmacovigilance and PML in the oncology setting. Cleve Clin J Med 78 (Suppl 2):S13–S17
2. Carson KR, Evens AM, Richey EA, Habermann TM, Focosi D, Seymour JF, Laubach J, Bawn SD, Gordon LI, Winter JN, Furman RR, Vose JM, Zelenetz AD, Mamtani R, Raisch DW, Dorshimer GW, Rosen ST, Muro K, Gottardi-Littell NR, Talley RL, Sartor O, Green D, Major EO, Bennett CL (2009) Progressive multifocal leukoencephalopathy after rituximab therapy in HIV-negative patients: a report of 57 cases from the Research on Adverse Drug Events and Reports project. Blood 113:4834–4840
3. Carson KR, Focosi D, Major EO, Petrini M, Richey EA, West DP, Bennett CL (2009) Monoclonal antibody-associated progressive multifocal leucoencephalopathy in patients treated with rituximab, natalizumab, and efalizumab: a Review from the Research on Adverse Drug Events and Reports (RADAR) Project. Lancet Oncol 10:816–824
4. Data on file (Genentech, Incorporated)
5. Calabrese LH, Molloy ES, Huang D et al (2007) Progressive multifocal leukoencephalopathy in rheumatic diseases: evolving clinical and pathologic patterns of disease. Arthritis Rheum 56:2116–2128
6. Boddy CS, Bennett CL, Norris LB, et al (2014) Rituximab-associated progressive multifocal leukoencephalopathy (PML) in HIV-negative patients: an updated report of 231 confirmed cases from the Southern Network on Adverse Reactions (SONAR)/Washington University collaboration (2000–2012). Presented at the 56th ASH Annual Meeting and Exposition in San Francisco, CA; December 6–9, 2014. ASH Abstract #4456. http://www.hematology.org/Annual-Meeting/

Charles L. Bennett MD, Ph.D., MPP, SmartState Chair and Frank P. and Josie M. Fletcher Chair of Medication Safety and Efficacy and Director, SmartState Center for Medication Safety and Efficacy, is also a Visiting Scholar at the City of Hope National Cancer Institute Designated Comprehensive Cancer Center in Duarte, California and is the co-editor of this book, Cancer Policy (2nd Edition). Dr. Bennett is a Phi Beta Kappa and High Honors graduate in mathematics from Swarthmore College, earned his medical degree in 1981 from the University of Pennsylvania Perelman School of Medicine, and completed internal medicine, hematology, and oncology training at the Michael Reese Hospital and the University of Chicago Pritzger School of Medicine before completing his Ph.D. and Masters in Public Policy degrees with honors in social science at the RAND Pardee Graduate School of Public Policy in Santa Monica, California. He has led a 20-year National Institutes of Health funded pharmacovigilance called the Research on Adverse Drug events And Reports (RADAR) and subsequently called to Southern Network on Adverse drug Reactions (SONAR) at the University of South Carolina College of Pharmacy.

Bartlett Witherspoon MBA is a third-year medical student at the Medical University of South Carolina and a graduate of Vanderbilt University's Masters in Business Administration program. He is an active co-investigator with Dr. Bennett and the SONAR project and has been a lead co-investigator on published manuscripts on fluoroquinolone-associated disability and on biosimilar oncology products.

Kenneth R. Carson MD, Ph.D. is Assistant Professor of Medicine at the Rush University School of Medicine and is also Vice-President for Tempus, Incorporated. He is a hematologist/oncologist trained at Northwestern University with a Ph.D. in public health from the University of Illinois at Chicago. He is a long-time collaborator with RADAR and SONAR and was the first author of the important 2009 manuscript in Blood describing 57 cases of rituximab-associated progressive multifocal leukoencephalopathy.

Maximum Accuracy Machine Learning Statistical Analysis—A Novel Approach

8

Shannon Ugarte, Paul Yarnold, Paul Ray, Kevin Knopf, Shamia Hoque, Matthew Taylor, and Charles L. Bennett

8.1 Introduction

Logistic regression is a statistical tool of paramount significance in the field of epidemiology [1] and ranks as one of the most frequently published multivariable analyses for designs involving a single binary dependent variable and one or more independent variables in the fields of public health [2, 3] and medical [4] research.

Studies of the quality of analytic and documentation aspects of articles using logistic regression report prevalent, important deficiencies in published research from the USA and Europe [5–7], China [8] and India [9]. A major source of model misspecification is failing to include crucial interactions among independent variables. Investigators report that statistical models which evaluate only main effects occurred in 50% to 96% of published research [1, 5–7]. Such model *misspecification* is problematic because omitting crucial interaction terms yields a suboptimal solution which fails to best explain the data [10–14]. Furthermore, omitting a crucial *mediating variable* from the model can induce paradoxical confounding vis-

S. Ugarte · P. Yarnold · P. Ray · K. Knopf · S. Hoque · M. Taylor · C. L. Bennett (✉)
SONAR (Southern Network on Adverse Reactions) Program, University of South Carolina
College of Pharmacy, Columbia, SC 29208, USA
e-mail: bennettc@cop.sc.edu

S. Ugarte
e-mail: shannonu1303@gmail.com

P. Yarnold
e-mail: paulyarnold@planetyarnold.com

K. Knopf
e-mail: kknopf@alamedahealthsystem.org

S. Hoque
e-mail: hoques@cec.sc.edu

M. Taylor
e-mail: matthew_taylor@brown.edu

à-vis pooling of disparate groups—for example, one group having high scores with another group having low scores [14–16].

The validity of *all linear models*, including logistic regression, requires satisfying three criteria.

1. First, *every variable* (and interaction term) in the model is important in classifying *every observation* in the sample. In contrast, using the nonlinear nonparametric methods discussed ahead, different variables and interaction terms may be used to classify different groups of observations in the sample: one set of variables and interactions may be used to classify one group, another set may be used to classify a different group, etc.
2. Second, every variable (and interaction) term in the linear model has an *identical direction of influence*, positively or negatively predictive, *for every observation* in the sample. In contrast, using the nonlinear nonparametric methods different variables and interaction terms may be positively, negatively, or non-predictive for different observation groups.
3. Third, every variable (and interaction term) in the linear model has an equivalent *magnitude of influence* for every observation in the sample. In contrast, using the nonlinear nonparametric methods variables may use different thresholds to define different sample partitions.

A practical limitation of all linear models is that every observation having missing data on any variable or interaction term used in the model is dropped from the analysis. In contrast, using the nonlinear nonparametric method only observations missing data on attributes and interaction terms specifically used to classify them are dropped from the analysis.

This chapter provides an example of how multivariable data from a large observational data set can be analyzed using the traditional statistical approach of logistic regression analysis, versus using modern nonlinear nonparametric approaches [16–20].

8.1.1 Data Analysis in Practice

Data herein are used to discriminate administration of use of two erythropoiesis stimulating agents in the settings of lung, colorectal, or breast cancer for patients in whom chemotherapy-induced anemia was developed. The drugs are shorter-acting (epoetin alfa) and longer-acting (darbepoetin) biologics which prevent the development of anemia among cancer patients who receive chemotherapy. Epoetin alfa received approval from the Food and Drug Administration (FDA) for this indication in 1991. Darbepoetin received FDA approval for this indication, but at a less frequent dosing interval, in 2002.

The dataset includes information on 37,702 persons with a diagnosis of cancer of the breast, colorectum, or lung who received epoetin alfa or darbepoetin prescriptions. Erythropoiesis stimulating agents are exogenous sources of the biologic hormone erythropoietin, which stimulates the production of red blood cells. It is important to note that unexpected, but important side effects of these drugs were discovered in 2004 and 2008. This discovery was accompanied by the manufacturer adding a warning to the product label in 2004 and a more stringent "Boxed Warning" to the product label in 2008. These warnings advised physicians that use of epoetin or darbepoetin was associated with significantly increased risks of cancer stimulation and death in the setting of cancer patients with chemotherapy-induced anemia. These safety concerns were particularly important, as the primary cancer indication for these two drugs is to prevent anemia from occurring among cancer patients with chemotherapy-induced anemia. Following the "warning" addition to the product label in 2004 and the more stringent "Box Warning" in 2008, physicians were increasingly aware that use of epoetin and darbepoetin in this setting could increase a cancer patient's risk of death. In 2011, the FDA expressed concern that the Boxed Warning was not being heeded by physicians and ordered the manufacturer to obtain patient and physician consent with each cancer patient before epoetin or darbepoetin was administered. This very stringent safety effort is known as a Risk Evaluation and Mitigation Strategy (REMS). It is extremely rare for the FDA to require patient and provider consent, and this only occurs in clinical settings where death or serious harm can occur following administration of a drug.

Historical data were obtained from the IMS LifeLink™ Health Plan Claims Database which contains fully adjudicated medical and pharmaceutical claims (inpatient/outpatient diagnoses and procedures, retail/mail-order prescription records, dates of service) for 71 million unique patients from 103 commercial managed care health plans across the US (16 million covered lives/year). Patients were included if they had a diagnosis of breast, colon, or lung cancer, and were excluded if they had a diagnosis of chronic kidney disease, dialysis, or other types of cancer besides the three target cancer types. Patient-level paid claims were extracted from 5/1/2004 (study start) to 12/31/2012 (study end).

Patient-level data elements used in analysis were date-specific paid claims including the following information: medication (epoetin, n = 1,338 patients; darbepoetin, n = 36,364 patients); cancer (breast, colorectal, or lung); age (years); gender; region of the country (East, South, Midwest, or West); time period (post the 2004 warning and prior to the 2008 Boxed Warning [5/1/2004–4/30/2008] = 2; post the 2008 Boxed Warning [5/1/2008–1/31/2010] = 3; post-REMS period [2/1/2010–12/31/2012] = 4); an index of the presence of comorbid medical illnesses (Charlson index); indicators of whether the patient received a blood transfusion or radiation therapy; and an indicator of the patient having a coded diagnosis of anemia in the claims file.

8.1.2 Logistic Regression (MELR) Analysis

For MELR discriminating the use of epoetin (group 1) versus darbepoetin (group 2), reference categories were used for cancer type and geographic region. Neither the coefficients for the comorbidity index, nor for contrasts of breast versus lung

Table 8.1 MELR results predicting epoetin versus darbepoetin use

| 95% CI bound | | | | | | |
Variable (attribute)	Coefficient	Std error	*P*<	OR	Lower	Upper
Period	−0.141	0.045	0.002	0.868	0.795	0.949
Cancer (breast vs. colon)	0.287	0.084	0.001	1.333	1.130	1.572
Cancer (breast vs. lung)	0.111	0.076	0.145	1.117	0.963	1.296
Anemia (no vs. yes)	1.104	0.063	0.001	3.017	2.666	3.414
Radiation (no vs. yes)	0.416	0.068	0.001	1.516	1.326	1.733
Transfusion (no vs. yes)	0.250	0.090	0.005	1.285	1.077	1.532
Region (east vs. south)	0.663	0.102	0.001	1.941	1.591	2.369
Region (east vs. midwest)	−0.074	0.101	0.463	0.929	0.763	1.131
Region (east vs. west)	1.919	0.125	0.001	6.813	5.333	8.703
Age	−0.014	0.003	0.001	0.986	0.981	0.991
Gender (no vs. yes)	0.354	0.080	0.001	1.425	1.219	1.665
Comorbidity score	0.020	0.015	0.183	1.020	0.990	1.051
Constant	2.730	0.210	0.001	15.331	10.167	12.120

cancer, or East versus Midwest region, were statistically significant (Table 8.1). Statistically significant *negative* model coefficients emerged for the three time periods (delimited by the warning in 2004, the Boxed Warning in 2004, and the REMS in 2011) and patient age—which best predicted *epoetin* use. Statistically significant *positive* coefficients emerged for contrasts of breast versus colon cancer, and for contrasts of East versus South and East versus Midwest region, and for positive responses for anemia, radiation, and/or transfusion.

Classifying (i.e., predicting the actual class membership status of) an observation using a MELR model is a two-step process.

1. In *step one,* the probability of group membership (p) is computed using the observation's responses to the attributes in Table 8.1 as input data for the MELR model (formulaically expressed regression models are also described as being "equations").
2. In *step two,* the standard threshold-based decision rule is used to classify each observation as being a member of group 1 or of group 2 based on their p score. Thus, an observation having $p \leq 0.50$ is predicted to be from group 1 (epoetin), and an observation having $p > 0.50$ is predicted to be from group 2 (darbepoetin).

Presently, when computed for all observations, p ranged between 0.724 and 0.998. Thus, the standard decision rule which is used to obtain predicted membership in group 1 versus group 2 based upon p resulted in *all observations* being predicted to have used darbepoetin, and in *no observations* being predicted to have used epoetin.

The MELR model thus achieved 100% accuracy in predicting the observations that used darbepoetin, but it achieved 0% accuracy in predicting the observations that used epoetin.

The mean accuracy achieved across class categories by a predictive model is *normed against chance* using the effect strength for sensitivity (ESS) index on which 0 represents the accuracy which is expected by chance; 100 represents perfect (errorless) accuracy; and values less than 0 represent accuracy which is worse than expected by chance (an ESS of -100 indicates perfect inaccuracy) [16, 17]. By convention ESS < 25 is considered a relatively weak model; ESS < 50 is a moderate model; ESS < 75 is a relatively strong model; ESS < 90 is a strong model; and ESS of 90 or greater is a very strong model [16].

For an application involving two class categories (e.g., darbepoetin and epoetin), ESS is computed as

$$ESS = [(\text{Mean \% Accuracy Across Class Categories} - - 50)/50] \times 100$$

In the present case, Mean % Accuracy Across Class Categories = (100 + 0) / 2 = 50, so

$$ESS = [(50 - - 50)/50] \times 100$$

$$ESS = (0/50) \times 100$$

$$ESS = 0$$

For this MELR model ESS = 0, which is exactly the level of classification accuracy expected to be achieved by chance. Therefore, the predictive accuracy achieved by the MELE solution is exactly equivalent to chance.

8.1.3   Using ODA to Maximize the Accuracy of the MELR Model

Optimal Discriminant (or Data) Analysis, abbreviated as ODA, was used to identify the cut-point on predicted p which optimized the ESS obtained by the MELR model [21–23]. The optimized MELR model was

$$\text{if predicted } p < 0.97010353 \text{ then predict epoetin use;}$$
$$\text{if predicted } p > 0.97010353 \text{ then predict darbepoetin use.}$$

This ODA model correctly classified 1,068 (79.8%) of the 1,338 patients who received epoetin, and 22,373 (61.5%) of 36,363 patients who received darbepoetin.

Therefore, mean accuracy achieved across classes is $(79.8 + 61.5)/2 = 141.3/2 = 70.65$. The maximized accuracy achieved by the MELR model is computed as

$$ESS = [(70.65 - -50)/50] \times 100$$

$$ESS = (20.65/50) \times 100$$

$$ESS = 41.30$$

This optimized logistic regression model thus yielded a moderate ESS = 41.3 in *training* (total sample) analysis.

The classification accuracy achieved by any algorithm is summarized using a "confusion table," as provided in Table 8.2 for the optimized MELR model.

Considering *sensitivity*, the model accurately classified approximately 4 in 5 (79.8%) actual epoetin prescriptions (50% accuracy is expected by chance for each class category), and 3 in 5 (61.5%) actual darbepoetin prescriptions. Considering *predictive value*, approximately 1 in 7 (14.1%) of model classifications of an epoetin prescription were correct versus 99 in 100 (98.8%) if darbepoetin was administered. The greatest "room for improvement" in this application clearly lies in more accurately predicting patients who were prescribed epoetin, whom the model incorrectly predicted as having been prescribed darbepoetin.

For an application involving two class categories, ESS is consistent with the Area Under the Curve (AUC) statistic computed in ROC analysis, in which AUC = 0.50 is the accuracy expected by chance, AUC = 1.0 is perfect accuracy, and $0 \leq$ AUC < 50 indicates accuracy which is worse than expected by chance. ODA thus maximizes AUC attained by MELR models [24].

The fourth axiom of novometric (Latin: *new measure*) theory—the state of the art in maximum-accuracy analysis, states that ESS for an analysis is properly assessed in cross-generalizability analysis, not in training analysis [20]. Presently, the model classification performance assessed using one-sample "leave one out" (LOO) jackknife cross-generalizability analysis [16] fell to ESS = 40.0 (still an effect of moderate strength): the model sensitivity for predicting patients receiving epoetin declined to 78.5%.

Table 8.2 Confusion table for optimized MELR model applied in training analysis

		Predicted prescription		
		Epoetin	Darbepoetin	Sensitivity
Actual	Epoetin	1,068	270	79.8
Prescription	Darbepoetin	13,990	22,373	61.5
	Predictive Value	14.1		98.8

8.1.4 Novometric CTA Models Explicitly Maximizing ESS

Novometric analysis [20] identifies all the statistically viable models which exist for a given sample, class variable, and set of independent variables, which vary as a function of precision (ESS) and parsimony (the number of sample strata, i.e., unique groups identified by the CTA model). This analysis renders model misspecification *impossible* since all possible models are identified [25].

In the present example, for novometric analysis cancer type and region were both treated as dummy-coded multicategorical attributes: in maximum-accuracy analyses, no reference variables are needed [26]. The exploratory alternative hypothesis is that the use of epoetin versus darbepoetin can be discriminated using the attributes [16, 21]. To facilitate cross-generalizability, all models were constrained to have identical ESS values in training and LOO validity analysis.

Analysis first discriminated group status by conducting ODA for each attribute considered separately. Table 8.3 summarizes ODA models identified for each attribute, all of which yielded statistically significant levels of predictive accuracy. Effects of moderate strength ($25 \leq$ ESS < 50) were identified for patients with a diagnosis of anemia, and for patients in the South and West *versus* East and Midwest regions of the country: both were positively predictive of darbepoetin use. All other effects were relatively weak (ESS < 25): post-Black Box warning and post-REMS periods (vs. post-FDA warning), lung cancer (vs. breast and colon

Table 8.3 Predicting use of epoetin versus darbepoetin using individual attributes

Covariate	ODA model	Correct Prediction (%)	P<	ESS	D
Period	If period = 2 predict epoetin If period = 3,4 predict darbepoetin	40.7 70.2	0.001	11.6	15.2
Cancer	If cancer = breast or colon predict epoetin If cancer = lung predict darbepoetin	69.8 33.4	0.034	3.2	60.5
Anemia	If no predict epoetin If yes predict darbepoetin	49.0 77.3	0.001	26.3	5.6
Radiation	If no predict epoetin If yes predict darbepoetin	72.9 45.3	0.001	18.2	9.0
Transfusion	If no predict epoetin If yes predict darbepoetin	87.4 19.8	0.001	7.3	25.4
Region	If region = east or midwest predict epoetin If region = south or west predict darbepoetin	56.2 71.2	0.001	27.4	5.3
Age	If age $\leq$ 59 years predict darbepoetin If age > 59 Years predict epoetin	57.8 51.2	0.001	9.6	18.8
Gender	If female predict epoetin If male predict darbepoetin	78.0 26.2	0.001	4.2	45.6
Comorbidity Score	If score $\leq$ 1 predict epoetin If score > 1 predict darbepoetin	16.8 92.4%	0.001	9.2	19.7

cancer), radiation, transfusion, male gender, age ≤ 59 years, and comorbidity score >1 predicted darbepoetin use.

ESS corrected for model complexity is assessed by the Distance (D) statistic which indicates the number of additional variables, each returning the mean ESS attained by the model, required to achieve perfect prediction [20]. The model having the lowest D statistic is most parsimonious [27].

ODA models evaluate the ability of each individual attribute to predict (discriminate) the class variable. In contrast, classification tree analysis (CTA) models identify subsets of different attributes, and/or multiple cut-points on individual attributes, that predict (discriminate) the class variable) [18, 19, 25]. The second and third axioms of novometric theory outline how to identify the descendant family: all statistically viable CTA models that exist for a given sample, class variable, and set of attributes [20, 25].

Table 8.4 summarizes all CTA models which exist in the sample. Complexity levels range between two- and seven-strata, arising from one- to six-node (i.e., strata) models, respectively. All models in Table 8.4 achieved LOO-stable classification accuracy of moderate strength ($25 \leq$ ESS < 50).

The model yielding greatest ESS in Table 8.4, offering the greatest *translational* (i.e., precision-forecasting) opportunity among all models, was obtained by the seven-strata model illustrated in Fig. 8.1. CTA models initiate with a root node, from which two or more branches emanate and lead to other nodes or to model endpoints. Branches indicate pathways through the tree, and all branches ultimately terminate in a model endpoint. The CTA algorithm determines the attribute subset and associated cutpoints (or rules for multicategorical attributes [26]), as well as

Table 8.4 Selected CTA models predicting epoetin *versus* darbepoetin use

Correct prediction					
Strata	Smallest Strata N	Epoetin (%)	Darbepoetin (%)	ESS	D
7	2,149	76.91	64.56	41.47	9.88
6	2,679	74.44	65.58	40.02	8.99
5	3,053	68.76	71.22	39.98	7.51
4	3,283	76.68	63.11	39.79	6.05
3	8,797	83.26	54.33	37.58	4.98
2	11,232	56.20	71.18	27.38	5.30

Table 8.5 Staging table for epoetin use

Stage	Anemia	Region	N	%	Odds
1	Yes	South, West	19,979	1.12	1:83
2	Yes	East, Midwest	8,797	5.21	1:18
3	No	–	8,926	7.35	1:13

Note N is number of observations in each stage, and % is the percent of observations using epoetin, also given as approximate odds (used epoetin)

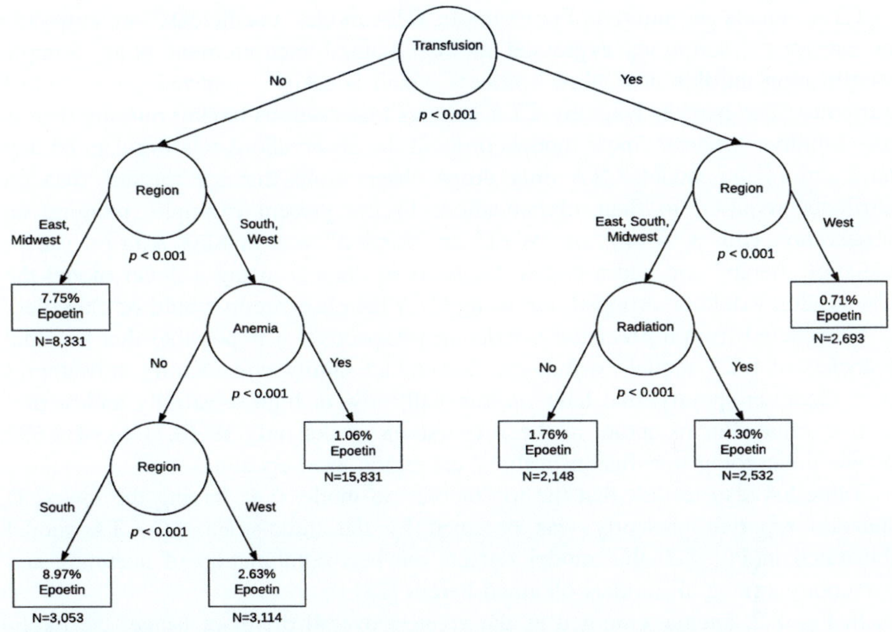

Fig. 8.1 Seven-strata CTA model predicting use of epoetin versus darbepoetin

attribute order within the model, which predicts the outcome with maximum accuracy (i.e., highest ESS, lowest D). Thus, CTA identifies a specific decision-making strategy which maximizes accuracy in predicting a specific outcome.

In this schematic illustration of the CTA model, circles are nodes, arrows are branches, and rectangles are model endpoints (strata). Numbers (or words if attributes are categorical) adjacent to arrows indicate the value of the cutpoint (category) for the node; the number underneath a node is generalized (per-comparison) p-value for the node; number of observations classified into each endpoint is indicated beneath the endpoint (rectangle); and percentage of observations having an epoetin prescription is given inside the endpoint.

Using CTA models to classify individual observations is straightforward. For example, consider a hypothetical patient who was transfused, lived in the South, and *did not* receive radiation therapy. Starting with the root node, the observation was transfused so the right branch is appropriate. Moving to the second node, since the observation lived in the South the left branch is appropriate. Finally, in the third node the observation did not receive radiation, so the left branch is appropriate: the hypothetical observation is thus classified into the strata for which 1.76% of 2,148 observations were prescribed epoetin. In this example, had the observation instead had radiation then the right-hand endpoint would be appropriate, a stratum for which 4.30% of 2.532 observations were prescribed epoetin.

CTA models are intuitive. For example, CTA model "coefficients" are cutpoints or category descriptions expressed in their natural measurement units. Sample stratification unfolds in a "flow" process which is easily visualized across model attributes. The manner whereby CTA handles observations having missing data is also intuitive: whereas linear models drop all the observations missing data on any attributes in the model, CTA only drops observations that are missing data on attributes required in their classification. In the present example, imagine an observation with a "score" of "West" on "Region" was missing data on use of radiation therapy and had a coded diagnosis of anemia: using a linear model the observation would be dropped, but using CTA the observation would be classified.

Considered from a *precision prediction* perspective, it is possible that terminal branches of CTA models within the descendant family will identify subsamples (i.e., model endpoints) that have an unusually low or high sensitivity and/or predictive value. For example, in the seven-strata model only 19 (0.71%) of 2,693 people undergoing transfusion in the West region used epoetin.

Table 8.4 also reveals that the top theoretical model (i.e., having the lowest D statistic) reported presently was obtained by the three-strata GO-CTA model illustrated in Fig. 8.2: this model reflects the best combination of accuracy and parsimony among all models obtained herein [27].

In Fig. 8.2, anemia emerged as the greatest overall driver of usage: the likelihood of epoetin (vs. darbepoetin) use is greatest among people who are negative for anemia. However, if positive for anemia, people receiving medical care in the East or Midwest regions of the USA (vs. the South or West regions) have a 5.21/1.12 or a 4.65-times greater likelihood of using epoetin.

While a *confusion table* summarizes the classification accuracy achieved by a model, a *staging table* sorts the model strata by ascending odds of class

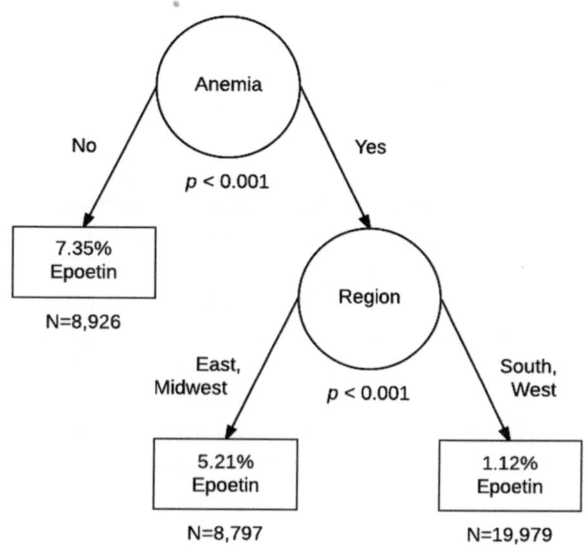

Fig. 8.2 Globally Optimal (GO) CTA model predicting epoetin versus darbepoetin use

membership. Table 8.5 is the staging table for the two-attribute, three-strata *globally optimal* CTA model—which has the lowest D statistic in this application and thus reflects the best combination of parsimony and predictive accuracy versus all other CTA models in the descendant family. Note that stage is an ordinal index of the likelihood of the patient being prescribed epoetin, whereas % is a more granular index (i.e., a real number having precision limited by N) ranging between 0 and 100%.

These results demonstrate three ubiquitous types of linear-model misspecifications which occur when estimating a MELR—all of which are circumvented by novometric CTA analysis. One misspecification is omission of underlying interactions from the model, thereby yielding a suboptimal ESS: here the 2-attribute CTA model had ESS = 37.58 (a moderate effect) versus ESS = 0 (a chance effect) for the 12-attribute MELR model. Beyond errors of *magnitude*, omitting interactions from linear models can induce *paradoxical confounding* whereby spurious effects are identified.

The second misspecification type is suboptimal construction of reference variables. Here, for the multicategorical attribute *region*, the reference variables in the MELR model separately compared South, West, and Midwest regions to the East. However, ODA and CTA models found other comparisons (see Figures) yielding greater ESS.

The third type of misspecification is relying on a single analytic model: reviews of published MELR analyses reported that only a fraction reported sensitivity analysis evaluating alternative models. In contrast, novometric analysis identifies all statistically viable maximum-accuracy models in the sample, and all these models may be directly compared with respect to accuracy normed against chance (ESS), and with respect to ESS normed against parsimony (D).

A commonly realized negative consequence of incorrectly specified linear models is their inability to identify theoretically meaningful findings. Obtaining the D statistic for the *optimized* MELR model identified presently, for example, requires computing the number of model "strata"—equal to the number of nodes (attributes) in the model plus one. The MELR model has nine binary and three ordered attributes, so number of strata = 12 + 1 = 13. For the optimized MELR model assessed in *training* analysis, $D = [100/(41.3/13)] - 13 = 18.5$—indicating that 18.5 additional attributes achieving the mean ESS obtained by the present model are needed to obtain perfect accuracy. For the optimized MELR model assessed in LOO *cross-generalizability* analysis, $D = [100/(40/13)] - 13 = 19.5$.

Such model misspecifications can yield substantively different findings obtained by MELR analysis versus novometric analysis. A heuristic method of assessing inter-method substantive agreement presently involves comparing MELR findings for individual attributes (sign of beta coefficient, *p*-value) versus ODA and/or CTA findings (direction indicated by ODA and/or CTA classification rules, *p*-values) for corresponding individual attributes. Presently, the MELR and ODA/CTA analyses agreed on direction of influence and statistical significance of most attributes; however the reference variables created for cancer type for MELR did not agree with the ODA assignment rule maximizing ESS. MELR identified a statistically significant difference between breast and colon cancer ($p < 0.001$), while ODA combined these cancers because they couldn't be discriminated. MELR found no difference between breast and lung cancer ($p < 0.145$), but ODA found a significant difference ($p < 0.034$). Also, comorbidity score had no statistically reliable coefficient in the MELR model, but ODA identified a statistically significant effect.

8.2 Conclusion

It is axiomatic that investigators should incorporate interactions and higher-order terms in (logistic) regression models in order to make them more robust (i.e., reduce the likelihood of potential model misspecification), researchers using traditional linear statistical methods must manually evaluate models involving different combinations of variables, interactions, and polynomials—without any guarantee that the best-fitting model will be identified [12]. In contrast, novometric analysis identifies every statistically viable model which exists for a sample, that explicitly maximizes model accuracy normed against chance (ESS). Obviously, identifying all maximum-accuracy models which exist for a sample precludes model misspecification [25].

The present exposition demonstrates the theoretical economy afforded by CTA models. For example, in the most complex 6-attribute 7-strata model (Fig. 8.1), the attribute *Region* appears three times: The CTA model involves only four unique attributes: *Transfusion* and *Region*—which apply to all observations in the sample, and *Anemia* and *Radiation*—which only apply to a portion of the observations in the sample—as a function of *Transfusion* status and USA *Region*.

Considered from theoretical and translational perspectives, a benefit of CTA models is that they clearly display how observations can transfer from one predicted class category to another—from category 0 to category 1, or vice versa. The subset of crucial attributes, critical threshold values, and possible pathways through the CTA model are easily visualized using novometric methods. This is not true for linear models. For example, for optimized MELR observations with predicted $p > 0.97010353$ are classified into class category 1 in this application. Determining how a given observation can transfer between class categories using a linear model requires identifying all variable combinations yielding predicted P values at or greater than this criterion, separately for every observation.

Considered from a precision prediction perspective, terminal branches of CTA models in the descendant family may identify subsamples (vis-à-vis model endpoints) with unusually high or unusually low prevalence of the class variable. In the seven-strata model, for example, only 19 (0.71%) of 2,693 people who underwent transfusion in the West region used epoetin. In a four-strata model branch, 14,708 (98.12%) out of 14,990 people who were positive for anemia *and* for radiation used darbepoetin. Exact discrete 95% (or any desired) confidence intervals may be constructed for all model-based estimates via Monte Carlo analysis [28].

Finally, considered from a causal inference perspective, ODA [29] and CTA-based matching techniques [30] provide additional dimensions and robustness to the analysis, versus what may be achieved using suboptimal methods.

This chapter supports prior research demonstrating that specifying logistic regression models using only main effects may often result in model misspecification. This chapter also illustrates how novometric analysis can be used to identify all the most accurate models—consisting of the most predictive variables and their interactions—which exist in the sample and vary as a function of complexity. Obtaining the descendant family of CTA models for the sample makes model misspecification impossible; clearly identifies model(s) having greatest translational application (maximum ESS); clearly identifies model(s) having greatest theoretical efficacy (minimum D); and clearly identifies model branches having outstanding precision-classification implications (high, LOO-stable predictive value). Investigators should therefore employ these modern tools with analogous analytic designs and in study design.

References

1. Ottenbacher KJ, Ottenbacher HR, Tooth LR, Ostir GV (2004) A review of two journals found that articles using multivariable logistic regression frequently did not report commonly recommended assumptions. J Clin Epidemiol 57:1147–1152
2. Hayat MJ, Powell A, Johnson T, Cadwell BL (2017) Statistical methods used in the public health literature and implications for training of public health professionals. PLoS ONE. https://doi.org/10.1371/journal.pone.0179032
3. Zardo P, Collie A (2014) Predicting research use in a public health policy environment: results of a logistic regression analysis. Implement Sci 9:142
4. Tetrault JM, Sauler M, Wells CK, Concato J. Reporting of multivariable methods in the medical literature. *Journal of Investigative Medicine 20–08; 56:* 954–957.
5. Kalil AC, Mattei J, Florescu DF, Sun J, Kalil RS (2010) Recommendations for the assessment and reporting of multivariable logistic regression in transplantation literature. Am J Transplant 19:1686–1694
6. Real J, Forne C, Roso-Llorach A, Martinez-Sanchez JM (2016) Quality reporting of multivariable regression models in observational studies. Medicine 95:e3653
7. Bagley SC, White H, Golomb BA (2001) Logistic regression in the medical literature: standards for use and reporting, with particular attention to one medical domain. J Clin Epidemiol 54:979–985
8. Zhang YY, Zhou XB, Wang QZ, Zhu XY (2017) Quality of reporting of multivariable logistic regression models in Chinese clinical medical journals. Medicine 96:e6972
9. Kumar R, Indiayan A, Chhabra P (2016) Evaluation of quality of multivariable logistic regression in Indian medical journals using multilevel modeling approach. Indian J Public Health 60:99–106
10. Wright RE. Logistic Regression. In LG Grimm, PR Yarnold (Eds.), *Reading and*
11. Understanding Multivariate Statistics (2005) Washington. APA Books, DC
12. Yarnold PR (1996) Discriminating geriatric and non-geriatric patients using functional status information: An example of classification tree analysis via UniODA. Educ Psychol Measur 56:656–667
13. Linden A, Yarnold PR (2016) Using data mining techniques to characterize participation in observational studies. J Eval Clin Pract 6:839–847

14. Linden A, Yarnold PR (2016) Using classification tree analysis to generate propensity score weights. J Eval Clin Pract 6:848–853
15. Linden A, Yarnold PR (2016) Identifying causal mechanisms in health care interventions using classification tree analysis. J Eval Clin Pract 6:854–858
16. Yarnold PR (1996) Characterizing and circumventing Simpson's paradox for ordered bivariate data. Educ Psychol Measur 56:430–442
17. Yarnold PR, Soltysik RC (2005) Optimal data analysis: Guidebook with software for Windows. APA Books, Washington, D.C.
18. Yarnold PR (2017) What is optimal data analysis? Optimal Data Analysis 6:26–42
19. Yarnold PR, Bryant FB (2015) Obtaining a hierarchically optimal CTA model via UniODA software. Optimal Data Analysis 4:36–53
20. Yarnold PR, Bryant FB (2015) Obtaining an enumerated CTA model via automated CTA software. Optimal Data Analysis 4:54–60
21. Yarnold PR (2017) What is novometric data analysis? Optimal Data Analysis 6:26–42
22. Yarnold PR, Soltysik RC (1991) Theoretical distributions of optima for univariate discrimination of random data. Decis Sci 22:739–752
23. Yarnold PR, Soltysik RC (1991) Refining two-group multivariable classification models using univariate optimal discriminant analysis. Decis Sci 22:1158–1164
24. Yarnold PR, Hart LA, Soltysik RC (1994) Optimizing the classification performance of logistic regression and Fisher's discriminant analyses. Educ Psychol Measur 54:73–85
25. Yarnold PR. UniODA vs. ROC analysis: Computing the "optimal" cut-point. *Optimal Data Analysis 2014*; *3*, 117–120.
26. Yarnold PR (2016) How many EO-CTA models exist in my sample, and which is the best model? Optimal Data Analysis 5:62–64
27. Yarnold PR (2013) Univariate and multivariate analysis of categorical attributes with many response categories. Optimal Data Analysis 2:177–190
28. Yarnold PR, Linden A (2016) Theoretical aspects of the D statistic. Optimal Data Analysis 5:171–174
29. Rhodes JN, Yarnold PR (2020) Generating novometric confidence intervals in R: Bootstrap analyses to compare model and chance ESS. Optimal Data Analysis 9:172–177
30. Linden A, Yarnold PR (2017) Minimizing imbalances on patient characteristics between treatment groups in randomized trials using classification tree analysis. J Eval Clin Pract 23:1309–1315
31. Linden A, Yarnold PR (2016) Combining machine learning and matching techniques to improve causal inference in program evaluation. J Eval Clin Pract 22:868–874

Shannon Ugarte MD is chief resident in internal medicine at Highland Hospital in Oakland, California and a 2022 Hematology/Oncology fellowship candidate. This is her first collaboration with SONAR under the guidance of Kevin B. Knopf, MD, MPH and Charles L. Bennett, MD Ph. D., MPP on cancer policy.

Paul Yarnold Ph.D. received his Ph.D. in academic psychology from the University of Illinois at Chicago, specializing in health psychology, measurement, and statistics. Paul was a Research (Full) Professor of Medicine (eight Divisional Affiliations) at Northwestern University Medical School; a Research (Full) Professor of Emergency Medicine at Northwestern University Medical School; and an Adjunct (Full) Professor of Psychology at the University of Illinois at Chicago. Presently he is an Adjunct (Full) Professor of Pharmacy at the University of South Carolina. Dr. Yarnold is an elected Fellow of the American Psychological Association (Quantitative and Qualitative Methods), and of the Society of Behavioral Medicine. Paul has published more than 600 journal articles and six books including two best-selling multivariate statistics texts, and he has a patent (cited in 1,280 later patents) for the first slot machine allowing user-input. His H-Index is 65, and he has close to 23,000 citations. He has been on editorial boards for six journals; served as compensated statistical reviewer for *Archives of Rehabilitation Medicine*; worked as Ad Hoc reviewer for more than 60 journals in the fields of medicine, psychology, biology, statistics, and engineering; and served as statistician on a DMC for a pharmaceutical company. He is a world-class big-game angler, a Level-3 Tripoli rocket scientist, a systems engineer, and he played the bass in a classic rock/classical blues band.

Paul Ray DO. FACOS is an Adjunct Professor University of South Carolina and a Clinical Adjunct Professor at Midwestern University in Downers Grove, Illinois. Dr. Ray received his master's degree based on research studying the protective mechanism action of taurine on ouabain infusions on the dog heart. This was his first publication in medical school, which he completed in 3 years and was also in the top 10% of his class. He continued publishing during his Urology residency at the University of Illinois. He became the second Osteopath admitted to any Allopathic Urology Residency program and to become Board Certified by the American Board of Urology. Shortly after finishing his Residency, he was appointed Chairman of Urology at Cook County Hospital.

Kevin Knopf MD is Division Chief of Hematology/Oncology at Highland Hospital in Oakland, California and Associate Professor at the University of South Carolina College of Pharmacy and a member of SONAR. He is Assistant Clinical Professor at University of California, San Francisco and a member of the Institute for Health Policy Studies at UCSF. He has expertise in health services research and decision analysis including cost effectiveness analysis and large-scale data analytics.

Shamia Hoque Ph.D., Associate Professor, Department of Civil Engineering, University of South Carolina and Principal Investigator for the American Cancer Society Institutional Research Grant on novel analytic approaches to identifying adverse drug reactions. She is a long-term co-investigator with Dr. Bennett and the SONAR project.

Matthew Taylor MD, MS is a first-year resident at the Brown University School of Medicine internal medicine program in Providence, Rhode Island. He has been an active collaborator under the guidance of Shamia Hoque, Ph.D. and Charles L Bennett, MD, Ph.D., MPP in the SONAR projects efforts to develop novel approaches to understanding adverse drug reactions.

Charles L. Bennett MD, Ph.D., MPP, SmartState Chair and Frank P. and Josie M. Fletcher Chair of Medication Safety and Efficacy and Director, SmartState Center for Medication Safety and Efficacy, is also a Visiting Scholar at the City of Hope National Cancer Institute Designated Comprehensive Cancer Center in Duarte, California and is the co-editor of this book, Cancer Policy (2nd Edition). Dr. Bennett is a Phi Beta Kappa and High Honors graduate in mathematics from Swarthmore College, earned his medical degree in 1981 from the University of Pennsylvania Perelman School of Medicine, and completed internal medicine, hematology, and oncology training at the Michael Reese Hospital and the University of Chicago Pritzger School of Medicine before completing his PhD and Masters In Public Policy degrees with honors in social science at the RAND Pardee Graduate School of Public Policy in Santa Monica, California. He has led a 20-year National Institutes of Health funded pharmacovigilance called the Research on Adverse Drug events And Reports (RADAR) and subsequently called to Southern Network on Adverse drug Reactions (SONAR) at the University of South Carolina College of Pharmacy.

Investigating Severe Adverse Reactions: Examples of the ANTICIPATE Methodology at Work

9

Charles L. Bennett and Shamia Hoque

9.1 Introduction

Severe adverse drug reactions (sADRs) are important causes of morbidity and mortality. The Southern Network on Adverse Drug Reactions (SONAR), a National Cancer Institute-funded pharmacovigilance program, has outlined a novel 9-stop methodology, termed ANTICIPATE, that has evaluated this methodology, among persons with chronic kidney disease (CKD). Examples of these sADRs include pure red-cell aplasia (PRCA), nephrogenic systemic fibrosis (NSF), and anaphylaxis. These four sADRs were identified and/or investigated by co-authors with SONAR and its National Cancer Institute-funded predecessor program, the Research on Adverse Drug Events and Reactions (RADAR) [1–10]. The initial description of ANTICIPATE has been with a single adverse drug reaction (ADR), peginesatide-associated pure red-cell aplasia (PRCA). Herein, we extend the ANTICIPATE methodology to four serious ADRS associated with CKD. We review root cause investigations and proposed strategies for toxicity eradication. The investigations were guided by ANTICIPATE and focused on signal detection, incidence estimation, causality identification, and toxicity eradication.

The ten-step framework, ANTICIPATE, was created to facilitate systematic analysis of four sADRs among chronic kidney disease (CKD) patients. It is a structured approach building on SONAR's work for general sADR evaluations [11]. SADRs were identified among CKD patients and were personally evaluated by SONAR and/or RADAR co-investigators: epoetin-associated PRCA (CLB, ICM, DC), HX575-associated PRCA (ICM), gadolinium-based contrast agents

C. L. Bennett · S. Hoque (✉)
SONAR (Southern Network on Adverse Reactions) Program, University of South Carolina College of Pharmacy, Columbia, SC 29208, USA
e-mail: hoques@cec.sc.edu

C. L. Bennett
e-mail: bennettc@cop.sc.edu

C. Bennett et al. (eds.), *Cancer Drug Safety and Public Health Policy*,
Cancer Treatment and Research 184, https://doi.org/10.1007/978-3-031-04402-1_9

(HST), and peginesatide-associated anaphylaxis (CLB, TH, ICM). Individually, these sADRs have been described in detail [1, 4, 6–10, 12, 13].

As outlined in our initial publication of ANTICIPATE, the framework consists of three items for signal detection (**A**wareness of toxicities, **N**otification of safety personnel, **T**alking with clinicians; four items for incidence estimation (**I**ncorporating simplicity into clinical settings; **C**omparing event rates from different settings; **I**nterim safety analyses; and **P**ilot clinical trial design for safety assessment); and three items for cause analyses/toxicity eradication recommendations (**A**ssessing a range of potential causes; **T**hinking outside the box; and **E**xperience counts).

Data sources for persons who have facilitated ANTICIPATE investigations include in-person visits with co-investigators; scientists at the Center for Biologic Evaluation and Research (CBER) and the Center for Drug Evaluation and Research (CDER) of the Food and Drug Administration (FDA); employees of the Danish Department of Health and the Danish Ministry of Health; employees in regulatory and clinical affairs at manufacturers of epoetin and darbepoetin and gadolinium-based contrast agents; family members of persons who developed one of the most serious ADRS (nephrogenic systemic fibrosis (NSF)); clinicians who treated NSF patients; epidemiologists, nephrologists, and hematologists who led studies of epoetin-associated PRCA in Canada; a clinician who led clinical trials of peginesatide; an investigator who led a phase 4 safety trial of peginesatide; a former executive of the original manufacturer of peginesatide; investigators affiliated with the International Center for NSF at Yale University in New Haven, Connecticut; and employees in clinical, regulatory, and legal affairs at a manufacturer for gadolinium-based contrast agents (GBCAs). Other data sources included publicly available documents on safety advisory meetings disseminated by regulatory agencies in the United States, Europe, and Denmark and Position Papers disseminated by the manufacturer of a gadolinium-based contrast agent.

9.1.1 The Toxicities

Epoetin-associated pure red-cell aplasia (PRCA): Since 1988, millions of CKD patients have received epoetin (recombinant erythropoietin) for the treatment of anemia. Between 1988 and 1998, antibody-associated pure red-cell aplasia was reported in three patients who had received epoetin. Between January 1998 and April 2004, a group (led by CLB) reported 175 cases of epoetin-associated PRCA associated with the Eprex formulation, 11 cases with the Neorecormon formulation (from ex-United States countries), and 5 cases with the Epogen formulation (from the United States) [4]. Half of the cases occurred in France, Canada, the United Kingdom, and Spain. Between 2001 and 2003, exposure-adjusted incidence was 18 cases per 100,000 patient-years for the Eprex formulation with polysorbate 80 as a stabilizer, 6 per 100,000 patient-years for the Eprex formulation with human serum albumin as the stabilizer, 1 case per 100,000 patient-years for Neorecormon, and 0.2 case per 100,000 patient-years for Epogen. After the peak incidence of Eprex-associated PRCA occurred in 2001, interventions designed in response to drug-monitoring programs worldwide resulted in a reduction of more than 80 percent in the PRCA incidence due to Eprex. The primary intervention was to restrict administration of the Eprex formulation to the intravenous versus the subcutaneous route.

9.1.2   HX575-Associated PRCA

One of us (ICM) investigated instances of HX575-associated PRCA that occurred in a phase III trial among anemic pre-dialysis patients that was assessing the safety, immunogenicity, and efficacy of subcutaneous administration of HX575, an epoetin biosimilar, versus first-generation epoetins [12]. Two patients in the HX575 group developed neutralizing antibodies to erythropoietin and clinical PRCA manifestations. Soluble tungsten was found in HX575 syringes, most likely derived from pins used to manufacture the syringes [14]. Spiking of epoetin alfa with sodium polytungstate or an extract of tungsten pins used to manufacture the syringes induced the formation of aggregates, dimers that were covalently linked by disulfide bonds as well as higher order aggregates. Sodium polytungstate had a strong denaturing effect on the protein. Removing tungsten from the pins used for injection was followed by no more HX575-associated PRCA cases.

9.1.3   Gadodiamide-Induced Nephrogenic Systemic Fibrosis

In 2006, a nephrology trainee in Austria reported five instances of a new syndrome, termed at that time nephrogenic fibrosing dermopathy [15]. Within months, nephrologists, radiologist, and dermatologist in Denmark identified 20 CKD patients with the new syndrome [13]. Shortly thereafter, systemic involvement was identified and the syndrome was renamed nephrogenic systemic fibrosis (NSF) [16]. Afterward, 1603 NSF patients were reported worldwide- with 93% of the cases reported from 60 hospitals in the USA and the rest primarily from two hospitals in Denmark [7]. The outbreak dated back to 1998, when the Danish Medicines Agency (DMA) had approved a non-ionic linear gadolinium-based contrast agent (GBCA), gadodiamide, for magnetic resonance imaging (MRIs) tests, and removed a contra-indication against administering GBCAs to persons with renal insufficiency. In 2002, radiologists at Herlev Hospital in Copenhagen began performing gadodiamide-enhanced magnetic resonance angiography scans of CKD patients. In 2006, Herlev clinicians (led by HST) reported that of 108 CKD patients at Herlev Hospital who had received gadodiamide-enhanced MRI, 20 developed probable NSF [7]. Radiologists voluntarily discontinued administering gadodiamide and no new NSF cases at Herlev Hospital developed subsequently. In 2007, the European Medicines Agency and the Danish Medicines Agency contra-indicated gadodiamide administration to CKD patients, and no new NSF cases in Denmark were subsequently diagnosed.

9.1.4 Peginesatide-Associated Anaphylaxis

In 2013, a large dialysis organization in the United States initiated a phase IV post-approval clinical trial of a third-generation erythropoiesis stimulating agent, peginesatide, an agent that had received FDA approval in March 2012 [1]. Over the next six months, two fatal anaphylaxis and five serious anaphylaxis events occurred, prompting a temporary discontinuation and a study redesign that prohibited administering intra venous peginesatide within one hour of any other intravenous medication. One month after restarting the revised study, on February 11 and 12, 2013, field staff reported three fatal cardiorespiratory arrests and two episodes of grade 4 anaphylaxis. No new patients began to receive peginesatide after February 12, pending analysis of the pilot initiative data. Between July 2012 and February 2013, a total of about 60,000 doses of peginesatide had been administered to 19,540 patients. Five patients had fatal anaphylaxis; 6 patients had grade 4 anaphylaxis; and 17 patients had grade 3 anaphylaxis. Symptoms of anaphylaxis began within minutes after administration of first dose of peginesatide. There were 1.4 anaphylaxis events per 1000 patients. Peginesatide was withdrawn from the market in February 2013, only a year after its marketing approval, primarily due to concerns of fatal and serious anaphylaxis.

9.2 The ANTICIPATE Evaluation

9.2.1 Signal Detection

Awareness of potential toxicities is important. Ten cases of PRCA following epoetin administration to CKD persons were published in 2000 by Casadevall et al. and heightened our focus on epoetins again being causal in the development of PRCA [17]. This awareness was key to identification of 181 cases of Eprex-associated PRCA in FDA's Adverse Event System (FAERS) database and subsequently identification of two cases of PRCA following administration of a biosimilar epoetin (HX575) in the clinical trial setting [6, 12]. Findings identifying fibrosis following exposure to unchelated gadolinium in mice were critical to recognition of gadolinium as the most likely cause of NSF in CKD patients, although this basic science discovery, known by the manufacturers in the 1980s, was uncovered by clinicians decades later during legal discovery procedures [18]. Anaphylaxis did not occur in pre-approval clinical trials involving 2,000 peginesatide-treated CKD patients [19–21]. The initial reporter of peginesatide-associated anaphylaxis first became aware of three cases of fatal anaphylaxis two months after the phase IV clinical trial of peginesatide had been discontinued [1].

Notify safety personnel rapidly about initial sADR occurrences. Manufacturers of three brands of epoetin were notified of 11 persons who developed epoetin-associated PRCA between 1998 and 1999 [17]. In 2011, clinical trial personnel were notified that two CKD patients participating in a double blind randomized clinical trial of subcutaneous administration of HX575 had developed PRCA [12]. In 2006, a nephrologist reported to the Danish Medicines Agency that 20 CKD persons had developed severe NSF shortly after undergoing an MRI with gadodiamide (a linear-chelated gadolinium-based contrast agent [7]. Nurses at four dialysis centers participating in a peginesatide post-approval clinical trial reported to study monitors that over a two-day period, three fatal and two near-fatal anaphylaxis events had occurred among five peginesatide-treated patients at four dialysis centers participating in a phase IV FDA mandated clinical trial [1].

Talk with field personnel about details of the initial sADRs. Field discussions led to the clarification that the toxicities were most likely product related, rather than class related. The hematologist in France who evaluated the initial PRCA cases reported that all 11 epoetin-associated PRCA cases had received one specific formulation of epoetin, the Eprex formulation—a formulation manufactured by Johnson and Johnson and marketed extensively in countries outside of the United States. Clinical personnel in the HX575 phase III trial reported that PRCA had begun following several months of subcutaneous administration of the biosimilar HX575 and that no PRCA cases had been identified in the control arms where branded epoetin was administered subcutaneously. In evaluating NSF, clinicians at Herlev Hospital in Copenhagen noted that all affected patients had received one specific gadolinium-based contrast agent product, gadodiamide, where the chelate is linear. They communicated this finding to Thomas Grobner, a nephrology medical trainee in Austria (who had reported the first cases of NSF a few months earlier associated with a different gadolinium-based contrast agent) [15]. Upon re-review by Grobner of the medical records of the patients he reported (at the request of Danish clinicians) his findings. It was discovered that the NSF patients in Austria as well as Denmark had all received the identical agent, gadodiamide and that the initial report from Austria had incorrectly implicated a different gadolinium-based contrast agent [7]. Nurses observing peginesatide administration at dialysis clinics involved in a phases IV safety trial reported to the FDA that death and anaphylaxis followed immediately after peginesatide administration and that in their clinical opinion, peginesatide was the only drug that was likely to be causally related [1].

Incorporate simplicity into clinical settings where sADRs are being evaluated. For Eprex-associated PRCA, after identifying initial cases of Eprex-associated PRCA, a collaboration of epidemiologists, nephrologists, and hematologists in Canada initiated a retrospective epidemiologic study of subcutaneous and intravenous administration of several branded epoetin formulations to CKD patients [22]. For HX575, clinical trial patients who received branded epoetin did not develop PRCA, allowing investigators to focus on HX575 as the most likely PRCA cause when two cases were identified. For gadolinium-associated NSF, radiologists postulated an association of NSF with gadodiamide, a contrast agent with a frail linear chelate which should protect the body from the toxic gadolinium, and switched to another agent with a less frail macrocyclic structure of the chelate [6, 7].

After becoming aware that anaphylaxis occurred shortly following intravenous administration of several medications to CKD patients (including peginesatide), the Peginesatide Monitoring Committee mandated a protocol revision that no other medication be administered within one hour of peginesatide [19].

9.3 sADR Data Analysis

Compare sADR numbers and rates from different settings. For antibody-mediated PRCA, incidence rates were 15 per 100,000 CKD patients with subcutaneous administration of Eprex versus < 5 per 100,000 CKD patients with subcutaneous or intravenous administration of other formulations [4, 5, 22]. For HX575, one randomized multi-center trial of 375 anemic pre-dialysis patients who received the product subcutaneously identified two cases of PRCA among HX575 patients versus none who received branded formulations of epoetin [12]. For NSF, clinician investigators at Herlev Hospital examined the skin of all patients who had undergone enhanced MRI, whereas clinician investigators at Skejby Hospital only looked at patient records. Both evaluations occurred after gadodiamide use had been discontinued for 4 years at the respective hospital. Clinical investigators in Copenhagen reported that among patients with stage 5 CKD, NSF rates were 18% at Herlev Hospital versus 4.7% at Skejby Hospital [7, 9, 10]. While each hospital had administered gadodiamide to a similar number of CKD patients, gadolinium had been administered to 88 CKD patients at Herlev Hospital with stage 5 CKD versus 17 CKD patients at Skejby Hospital with stage 5 CKD when they underwent MRIs (only some of which developed NSF) [9, 10]. (NSF develops almost exclusively among patients with stage 5 CKD (estimated glomerular filtration rate <15 ml/min/1.73m^2 or on dialysis) [6, 7]. There were 10 peginesatide-associated fatal anaphylaxis events in the post-approval phase IV study including 19,540 CKD patients [1, 19].

Interim data analyses of clinical trials or a consecutive case series should be conducted. For PRCA, an interim epidemiologic report in Canada identified PRCA rates of 270 per million CKD patient years who received epoetin formulated with polysorbate 80 subcutaneously versus <10 per million CKD patient years who received that product intravenously and versus all other epoetin products administered subcutaneously or intravenously [22]. The manufacturer of HX575 reported that interim analyses of phase III clinical trial data identified two instances of antibody-mediated PRCA with HX575 administration versus no instances with epoetin administration (necessitating early study closure) [12, 14]. For gadolinium-based contrast agent associated NSF, an interim case identification conducted by the Danish Department of Health analysis identified 10 cases of NSF, two of which were associated with gadodiamide, a linear-chelated and one of which reportedly had not undergone MRI testing [7]. The Peginesatide Monitoring Committee conducted an interim analysis in February 2013, identifying five instances of fatal anaphylaxis events following peginesatide administration.

Pre-approval and post-approval safety studies should be implemented. It was hypothesized that Eprex-associated PRCA could be eliminated by administering the product solely by the intravenous route [4]. After this change was carried out, a follow-up study found PRCA incidence following intravenous administration was similar to that for comparator ESAs [4]. For the HX575 epoetin biosimilar formulation, no additional PRCA cases were detected after glass syringes with high levels of tungsten in the plunger of the vial were withdrawn [12, 14]. For gadolinium, no additional NSF cases were detected after radiologists at Herlev Hospital in Copenhagen replaced the linear gadodiamide with a macrocyclic agent [8, 23]. Without the phase IV clinical trial evaluating the safety and efficacy of peginesatide in 348 dialysis centers, years may have passed before anaphylaxis following peginesatide administration was identified.

9.3.1 Root Cause Analyses/Toxicity Eradication

Assess a range of causes. For Eprex-associated PRCA, early theories focused on breaches in cold chain storage and supply chain management. Later theories focused on leachates that appeared to form in response to exposure to polysorbate 80-Eprex complexes. Another theory is that subcutaneous administration is more immunogenic than intravenous administration [4, 5]. For the biosimilar epoetin HX575-associated PRCA, soluble tungsten derived from pins used to manufacture glass syringes appeared to be causal [12, 14]. Spiking of epoetin alfa with sodium polytungstate or an extract of tungsten pins used to manufacture HX575-containing glass syringes induced aggregate formation [14]. These aggregates were dimers linked by disulfide bonds and higher-order aggregates. Sodium polytungstate had a strong denaturing affect. Another causal factor was the administration route, as Eprex-associated PRCA and HX575-associated PRCA only occurred with subcutaneous administration [4, 5]. For gadolinium-associated NSF, assessed causal factors included administration of gadolinium-based products, where the gadolinium ion was bound by a non-ionic linear chelate that allowed transmetallation of the gadolinium (with zinc, for example) [13]. NSF was not seen after administration of agents where the gadolinium ion was bound by a macrocyclic chelate. This toxicity was identified in patients on dialysis. Renal insufficiency results in contrast agents remaining a long time in vivo whereas patients with normal renal function readily clear gadolinium agents [6, 7]. Other causal factors included pro-inflammatory states and high cumulative gadolinium dosing [6, 7]. For peginesatide, initial studies by the FDA and the manufacturer focused on supply chain management, cold storage, and manufacturing production—as anaphylaxis had not been observed in pre-approval clinical trials,

Think outside the box [24, 25]. Manufacturing decisions appear to be central to development of these sADRs. These included exchanging albumin with polysorbate 80 as a stabilizer of Eprex [4]; manufacturing ready-to-fill glass epoetin-HX575 syringes with a process that resulted in high residual tungsten levels in syringes [12, 14]; use of linear-chelated GBCAs (where the risk of liberation of the toxic gadolinium ion is significantly greater versus macrocyclic GBCAs); and adding phenol to multi-dose peginesatide vials as a preservative [26, 27].

Experience counts. One hematologist and one nephrologist with experience in sADRs and erythropoietins (CLB and ICM, respectively) were central to the Eprex-associated PRCA investigations [4, 5, 20, 21, 28]. The nephrologist (ICM) with expertise in HX575 and PRCA evaluated peginesatide-associated PRCA [5, 20, 21, 28]. The nephrologist (ICM) also had extensive experience with epoetin biosimilars which facilitated the evaluation of HX575-associated PRCA. A nephrology trainee (PM) identified the first twenty cases of gadolinium-based contrast agent induced NS [13]. A radiologist (HST) identified the likely basic science rationale, the epidemiology of the toxicity, the improved safety profiles when other GBCAs were administered and issued guidelines to avoid NSF [7]. A hematologist with extensive experience in sADR evaluation of epoetins (CLB) led the evaluation of peginesatide-associated anaphylaxis [1].

9.4   Conclusion

Overall, the ANTICIPATE framework guided our reporting of four sADRs among CKD patients as well as eradication strategies. In interpreting our findings, several factors should be considered.

Awareness of unique events as being a new safety signal requires "prepared minds." [24] For Eprex, the occurrence of PRCA was initially recognized and reported by Casdevall et al., and then two years elapsed before two independent follow-up analyses identified 181 instances of the same toxicity based on FDA data review as well as a review of cases in Canada based on a nation-wide epidemiologic survey [4, 22]. In each instance, awareness of the potential for PRCA to occur was critical as CKD patients are often very ill and have comorbid illnesses and transfusion-dependent anemia may not be worked up in many settings. For HX575, clinical investigators were very aware at this point of the potential for PRCA events to occur with a biosimilar epoetin, although none had been reported previously, and prospective monitoring of serum antibodies rapidly facilitated the identification of PRCA events in two individuals. For gadolinium-associated NSF at Herlev Hospital, the syndrome first occurred in 1998 and by 2005, the nephrologists had recognized 11 individuals with dermatopathic fibrosis syndrome- and requested epidemiologic assistance from the Danish Department of Health [7]. The association of the syndrome was delayed when the Department of Health review initially identified gadolinium administration in two patients [7]. Subsequent evaluation identified that a linear-chelated gadolinium-based contrast agent had been administered to all of the initially reported patients [7]. For peginesatide, four clinical trial nurses were extremely vigilant and were the first to associate peginesatide administration with anaphylaxis, despite co-administration of several other medications around the time of peginesatide administration [1].

Efficient communications, in some cases augmented by political discussions, with national regulatory agencies, clinical trial coordinating centers, or the Department of Health facilitated clarification of safety signals and toxicity eradication. Casaedevall et al. [29], our group, and the Canadian group communicated PRCA findings to the three manufacturers of epoetins and regulatory agencies in the United States, Canada, and Europe. Subsequently, the regulatory agencies declared that subcutaneous administration of the Eprex formulation with polysorbate 80 was contra-indicated. For HX575-associated PRCA, as soon as two cases of PRCA were identified, the clinical trial was halted and toxicology studies identified tungsten contamination of the product syringes [14, 30]. A restart with a different syringe facilitated a successful completion of the study trial. For NSF, warnings about linear-chelated GBCAs as a probable cause of NSF as noted by clinicians at Herlev Hospital in Copenhagen were not disseminated by the Department of Health until four years had passed, and additional gadodiamide-associated NSF cases at Skejby Hospital were noted [7]. The delayed decision to disseminate a product warning was viewed by many as a political decision. For peginesatide, close collaboration of clinical trial investigators, the manufacturer, and FDA scientists facilitated identification of phenol as the most likely causal agent. Basic science studies conducted by FDA scientists ruled out complement activation as a possible cause, although this pathway was causal in the FDA's previous investigation of anaphylaxis occurring among CKD patients who received contaminated heparin [26, 31].

Toxicity eradication is the cornerstone of drug safety initiatives. For three sADRs, Eprex-associated PRCA, HX575-associated PRCA, and gadodiamide-associated NSF, product-specific versus class-specific causes were identified. For Eprex-associated PRCA and HX575-associated PRCA, changes in the manufacturing processes were critical. For gadodiamide-associated NSF, a strategy of using other products in the class was developed and no new NSF cases (when these contrast medium products were used (after 2009)) have been reported subsequently. For peginesatide-associated anaphylaxis, a proposed strategy of using single unit vials without preservatives continues to be under consideration by the manufacturer but has not been implemented at this time.

In conclusion, the ANTICIPATE framework has facilitated our review of the identification, evaluation, and potential toxicity eradication of four sADRS occurring among CKD patients. Going forward, this method should be evaluated in other settings.

References

1. Bennett CL, Jacob S, Hymes J, Usvyat LA, Maddux FW (2014) Anaphylaxis and hypotension after administration of peginesatide. N Engl J Med 370:2055–2056
2. Jacob S, Nichols P, Macdougall IC, Qureshi Z, Chen B, Yant g YT (2018) Investigating serious adverse drug reactions in patients receiving erythropoiesis stimulating agents: a root cause analysis using the ANTICPATE framework. Am J Ther; e670–e674

3. European Medicines Agency (2014) Pharmacovigilance Department. One-year report on human medicines pharmacovigilance tasks of the European Medicines Agency. May 20, 2014. Accessed 25 March 2019

4. Bennett CL, Luminari S, Nissenson AR, Tallman MS, Klinge SA, McWilliams N, McKoy JM, Kim B, Lyons EA, Trifilio S, Raisch DW, Evens AM, Kuzel TM, Schumock GT, Belknap SM, Locatelli F, Rossert J, Casadevall N (2004) Pure red-cell aplasia and epoetin Therapy. New Engl J Med 351:1403–1408

5. Macdougall IC, Casadevall N, Locatelli F, Combe C, London GM, Di Paolo S, Kribben A, Fliser D, Messner H, McNeil J, Stevens P, Santoro A, De Francisco AL, Percheson P, Potamianou A, Foucher A, Fife D, Mérit V, Vercammen E (2015) PRIMS study group. Nephrol Dial Transpl 30:451–460

6. Bennett CL, Starko KM, Thomsen HS, Cowper S, Sartor AO, MacDougall I, Qureshi ZP, Bookstaver PB, Miller AD, Norris LB, Xirasagar S, Trenery A, Lopez I, Kahn A, Murday A, Luminari S, Cournoyer D, Locatelli F, Ray P, Mattison DR (2012) Linking drugs to obscure illnesses: lessons from pure red cell aplasia, nephrogenic systemic fibrosis, and Reye's syndrome. A report from the SOuthern Network on Adverse Reactions (SONAR). J Genl Intern Med 27:1697–1703

7. Bennett CL, Qureshi ZP, Sartor AO, Norris LB, Murday A, Xirasagar S, Thomsen HS (2012) Gadolinium induced nephrogrenic systemic fibrosis, the rise and fall of an iatrogenic disease. Clin Kidney J 5:82–88

8. Elmholdt TR, Olesen AB, Jørgensen B, Kvist S, Skov L, Thomsen HS, Marckmann P, Pedersen M (2013) Nephrogenic systemic fibrosis in Denmark—a nationwide investigation. PLoS ONE 8(12):e82037. https://doi.org/10.1371/journal.pone.0082037

9. Elmholdt TR, Pedersen M, Jorgensen B, Sondergaard K, Jensen JD et al (2011) Nephrogenic systemic fibrosis is found only among gadolinium-exposed patients with renal insufficiency: a case-control study from Denmark. Br J Dermatol 165:828–836. https://doi.org/10.1111/j.1365-2133.2011.10465.x[doi]

10. Rydahl C, Thomsen HS, Marckmann P (2008) High prevalence of nephrogenic systemic fibrosis in chronic renal failure patients exposed to gadodiamide, a gadolinium-containing magnetic resonance contrast agent. Invest Radiol 43:141–144. https://doi.org/10.1097/RLI.0b013e31815a3407[doi];00004424-200802000-00007

11. Bennett CL, Nebeker JR, Lyons EA, Samore MH, Feldman MD, McKoy JM, Carson KR, Belknap SM, Trifilio SM, Schumock GT, Yarnold PR, Davidson CJ, Evens AM, Kuzel TM, Parada JP, Cournoyer D, West DP, Sartor O, Tallman MS, Raisch DW (2005) The Research on Adverse Drug Events and Reports (RADAR) project. JAMA 293:2131–2140

12. Haag-Weber M, Eckhardt K-U, Horl WH, Roger SD, Vetter A, Roth K (2012) Safety, immunogenicity, and efficacy of a subcutaneous biosimilar epoetin-alfa (HX575) in non-dialysis patients with renal anemia: a multi-center randomized double-blind study. Clin Nephrol 77:8–17

13. Marckmann P, Skov L, Rossen K, Dupont A, Damholt MB, Heaf JG, Thomsen HS (2006) J Am Soc Nephrol 17:2359–2362

14. Seidl A, Richter M, Fischer R et al (2012) Tungsten-induced denaturation and aggregation of epoetin alfa during primary packaging as a cause of immunogenicity. Pharm Res 29:1454–1467

15. Grobner T (2006) Gadolinium—a specific trigger for the development of nephrogenic fibrosing dermopathy and nephrogenic systemic fibrosis? Nephrol Dial Transpl 21:1104–1108

16. Introcaso CE, Hivnor C, Cowper S, Werth VP (2007) Nephrogenic fibrosing dermopathy/nephrogenic systemic fibrosis: a case series of nine patients and review of the literature. Int J Dermatol 46(5):447–452

17. Casadevall N, Nataf J, Viron B, Kolta A, Kiladjian JJ, Martin-Dupont P, Michaud P, Papo T, Ugo V, Teyssandier I, Varet B, Mayeux P (2002) Pure red-cell aplasia and antierythropoietin antibodies in patients treated with recombinant erythropoietin. N Engl J Med 346:469–475

18. Hermanson T, Bennett CL, Macdougall IC (2016) Peginesatide for the treatment of anemia due to chronic kidney disease - an unfulfilled promise. Expert Opin Drug Saf 15(10):1421–1426. https://doi.org/10.1080/14740338.2016.1218467

19. Withdrawal assessment report for Omontys. European Medicines Agency. http://www.ema.europa.eu/docs/en_GB/document_library/Application_withdrawal_assessment_report/2013/09/WC500148933.pdf. Accessed 25 March 2019

20. Macdougall IC, Provenzano R, Sharma A, Spinowitz BS, Schmidt RJ, Pergola PE, Zabaneh RI, Tong-Starksen S, Mayo MR, Tang H, Polu KR, Duliege AM, Fishbane S, PEARL Study Groups (2013) Peginesatide for anemia in patients with chronic kidney disease not receiving dialysis. N Engl J Med 368(4):320–332. https://doi.org/10.1056/NEJMoa1203166

21. Fishbane S, Schiller B, Locatelli F, Covic AC, Provenzano R, Wiecek A, Levin NW, Kaplan M, Macdougall IC, Francisco C, Mayo MR, Polu KR, Duliege AM, Besarab A; EMERALD Study Groups. Peginesatide in patients with anemia undergoing hemodialysis. N Engl J Med. 2013 Jan 24;368(4):307–19. https://doi.org/10.1056/NEJMoa1203165.

22. Cournoyer D, Toffelmire EB, Wells GA, Barber DL, Barrett BJ, Delage R, Forrest DL, Gagnon RF, Harvey EA, Laneuville P, Patterson BJ, Poon MC, Posen GA, Messner HA, Canadian PRCA Focus Group (2004) Anti-erythropoietin antibody-mediated pure red cell aplasia after treatment with recombinant erythropoietin products: recommendations for minimization of risk. J Am Soc Nephrol 15:2728–2734

23. Elmholdt TR et al (2013) Nephrogenic system fibrosis in Denmark—a nationwide investigation. PLoS ONE 12:e82307

24. Trontell A (2004) Expecting the unexpected—drug safety, pharmacovigilance, and the prepared mind. N Engl J Med 351:1385–1387

25. Wood AJ (2000) Thrombotic thrombocytopenic purpura and clopidogrel—a need for new approaches to drug safety. N Engl J Med 342:1824–1826

26. Weaver JL, Boyne M, Pang E, Chimalakonda K, Howard KE (2015) Nonclinical evaluation of the potential for mast cell activation by an erythropoietin analog. Toxicol Appl Pharmacol pii:S0041–008X(15)30017-X. https://doi.org/10.1016/j.taap.2015.06.009. [Epub ahead of print]

27. Zhou Z, Bupp S, Kozlowski A (2015) Developing in vitro and in vivo models to predict drug-induced acute allergic reactions. Proceedings of the 2015 FDA science forum on emerging technologies. Bethesda, Maryland. http://www.fda.gov/downloads/ScienceResearch/AboutScienceResearchatFDA/UCM447461.pdf. Accessed 15 Jun 2022

28. Macdougall IC, Rossert J, Casadevall N, Stead RB, Duliege AM, Froissart M, Eckardt KU (2009) A peptide-based erythropoietin-receptor agonist for pure red-cell aplasia. N Engl J Med 361(19):1848–1855. https://doi.org/10.1056/NEJMoa074037

29. Casadevall N, Nataf J, Viron B, Kolta A, Kiladjian JJ, Martin-Dupont P, Michaud P, Papo T, Ugo V, Teyssandier I, Varet B, Mayeux P (2002) Pure red-cell aplasia and antierythropoietin antibodies in patients treated with recombinant erythropoietin. N Engl J Med 346(7):469–475

30. Macdougall IC, Roger SD, de Francisco A, Goldsmith DJ, Schellekens H, Ebbers H, Jelkmann W, London G, Casadevall N, Hörl WH, Kemeny DM, Pollock C (2012) Antibody-mediated pure red cell aplasia in chronic kidney disease patients receiving erythropoiesis-stimulating agents: new insights. Kidney Int 81(8):727–732. https://doi.org/10.1038/ki.2011.500. Epub 2012 Feb 15

31. Kishimoto TK, Viswanathan K, Ganguly T et al (2008) Contaminated heparin-associated with adverse clinical events and activation of the contact system. N Engl J Med 358:2457–2467

Charles L. Bennett MD, Ph.D., MPP, SmartState Chair and Frank P. and Josie M. Fletcher Chair of Medication Safety and Efficacy and Director, SmartState Center for Medication Safety and Efficacy, is also a Visiting Scholar at the City of Hope National Cancer Institute Designated Comprehensive Cancer Center in Duarte, California and is the co-editor of this book, Cancer

Policy (2nd Edition). Dr. Bennett is a Phi Beta Kappa and High Honors graduate in mathematics from Swarthmore College, earned his medical degree in 1981 from the University of Pennsylvania Perelman School of Medicine, and completed internal medicine, hematology, and oncology training at the Michael Reese Hospital and the University of Chicago Pritzger School of Medicine before completing his Ph.D. and Masters In Public Policy degrees with honors in social science at the RAND Pardee Graduate School of Public Policy in Santa Monica, California. He has led a 20-year National Institutes of Health funded pharmacovigilance called the Research on Adverse Drug events And Reports (RADAR) and subsequently called to Southern Network on Adverse drug Reactions (SONAR) at the University of South Carolina College of Pharmacy.

Shamia Hoque Ph.D., Associate Professor, Department of Civil and Environmental Engineering, University of South Carolina and Principal Investigator for the American Cancer Society Institutional Research Grant on novel analytic approaches to identifying adverse drug reactions. She is a long-term co-investigator with Dr. Bennett and the SONAR project.

Consequences to Patients, Clinicians, and Manufacturers When Very Serious Adverse Drug Reactions Are Identified (1997–2019): A Qualitative Analysis from the Southern Network on Adverse Reactions (SONAR)

Courtney R. Lubaczewski, Nancy F. Olivieri, William R. Hrushesky, and Charles L. Bennett

10.1 Introduction

Adverse drug/device reactions (ADRs) serious enough to lead to box warnings on drug labels or drug withdrawals occur in about one fifth of all new molecular entities [1]. They can result in patient harm, affect the careers of clinicians who report these toxicities, result in substantial costs and harms to patients, and lead to large revenue losses by manufacturers. We operationally define very serious ADRs based on serious toxicity (as defined by the Common Toxicity Criteria Adverse Events scale) that follow use of drugs or devices with publicly reported $1 billion dollars in sales and/or have either a publicly reported financial safety-related payments totaling $1 billion and/or have a publicly report clinical measure of serious toxicity or death from the ADR of 1000 or more persons.

This study follows our report on implications of publishing serious hematology and oncology ADRs by clinicians [2]. Most of these ADR publications were followed by addition of Boxed warnings to product labels. Boxed warnings are the most serious warning that can be added to product labels. Careful observation by clinicians of persons who received hematology and oncology drugs and then developed unexpected syndromes led to identification of fourteen serious ADRs. As the relevant ADR had not been published previously in the literature, these clini-

C. R. Lubaczewski · N. F. Olivieri · W. R. Hrushesky · C. L. Bennett (✉)
SONAR (Southern Network on Adverse Reactions) Program, University of South Carolina College of Pharmacy, Columbia, SC 29208, USA
e-mail: bennettc@cop.sc.edu

C. R. Lubaczewski
e-mail: lubaczec@email.sc.edu

N. F. Olivieri
e-mail: nancy@hemoglobal.org

© The Author(s), under exclusive license to Springer Nature Switzerland AG 2022
C. Bennett et al. (eds.), *Cancer Drug Safety and Public Health Policy*,
Cancer Treatment and Research 184, https://doi.org/10.1007/978-3-031-04402-1_10

cians were felt to be the persons most responsible for ADR identification. The study found that 83% of the fourteen clinicians reported experiencing negative feedback from manufacturers, half reported receiving negative feedback from universities or colleagues, and a third received negative feedback from regulatory officials [2].

We report on impacts of very serious ADRs identified between 1997 and 2019 on patients, clinicians who reported these events, and manufacturers of scrutinized drugs or devices. We extend our prior findings on hematologic and oncologic ADRs reporting to very serious ADRs. Our objective is to determine if previous accounts of physician, academic, and pharmaceutical impacts occurring after serious ADRs were published can be corroborated and better characterized.

10.2 Methods

The Southern Network on Adverse Reactions (SONAR) consists of co-investigators at fifty medical universities who have assisted with one or more evaluations of serious ADRs as part of two National Institutes of Health funded pharmacovigilance grants (1998–2010 and 2012–current). Co-investigators and faculty collaborators of the coinvestigators were queried about drugs or devices which satisfied the following criteria: the identified drug had large sales (generally at $100 million per year annually, but wide latitude was allowed); a clinician of whom they were aware had been the first author on the related manuscript describing a case series of a very serious ADR (operationally defined as severe organ failure or death) associated with that drug; large numbers of persons were injured as a result of the very serious ADR; and there had been some consideration that the drug might be withdrawn because of safety concerns. This search methodology formed the basis for clinicians to include in our qualitative analysis. Our main objective was to report on the personal and professional costs of publishing a manuscript describing a very serious ADR. We also evaluated events that occurred to the patients with the identified very serious ADR and to the pharmaceutical manufacturer of the implicated drug or device. The SONAR co-investigators and associated collaborators included many of the most prominent pharmacovigilance investigators in the country. Several of these individuals had testified on pharmaceutical safety before Congressional or Senate hearings on drug safety in hearings that focused on some of the drugs included in this qualitative study.

Overall, using the non-systematic approach for identification of drugs associated with very serious ADRs, SONAR identified 23 drugs and 2 devices in which rescinding of FDA marketing approval had been considered and a clinician collaborator had a primary role in uncovering these ADRs [3]. We reviewed titles and abstracts of FDA Advisory Committee meeting convened between 1997 and 2019 for meetings that focused on these drugs and devices. We searched for drugs or devices with the following characteristics: FDA Advisory Committee meeting advisors were asked to vote on recommending rescinding FDA approval for the drug or device; the initial ADR reporter was a physician who either treated persons with the relevant drug or persons who experienced the relevant toxicity and who was either the first or senior author on the ADR report; the implicated drug had publicly reported lifetime sales of $1 billion; publicly reported $1 billion in patient harm payments cited in one of the five highest US circulation newspapers (New York Times, Wall Street Journal, Chicago Tribune, Los Angeles Times, and USA Today) and had public reports of 1000 or more persons who had developed severe toxicities. Fifteen drugs and one device were included. Eight drugs and one device were excluded, although they were associated with severe ADRs. These included deferiprone, rituximab, brentuximab vedotin, lenalidomide, and thalidomide (no FDA Advisory Committee meetings were convened to address whether FDA approval should be rescinded); and peginesatide, ciprofloxacin, gemtuzumab ozogamycin, and vaginal morcellators (sales for each drug or device were less than $1 billion).

10.3   Results

Clinician reporting of serious ADRs resulted in negative consequences for clinicians, patients, and manufacturers. Between 1997 and 2019, eighteen clinicians in our sample had reported twenty very serious ADRs. FDA Advisory Committee hearings for these toxicities focused on whether the FDA should remove marketing approval. All twenty ADRs were reviewed at least one FDA Advisory Committee meeting. Eight hearings of committees of the United States House of Representatives or Senate queried whether manufacturers delayed in their reporting of serious ADRs. The toxicities that were evaluated included venous thromboembolism, cardiovascular events, tumor progression, jaw osteonecrosis, severe hypertension, cardiac valvulopathy, severe renal insufficiency, hemorrhagic stroke, drug-associated mortality, renal failure, severe neuropsychiatric toxicities, nephrogenic systemic fibrosis, and prosthetic hip failure. All but two of the ADRs were reviewed by government agencies in ex-United States countries. Almost all of the committees agreed with each other.

Safety signals were identified in several types of data sources: eight Phase III pharmaceutical funded clinical studies, one Phase III safety-focused clinical study, one case–control epidemiologic analysis, one case series, one meta-analytic effort, two registry focused analyses, and a comprehensive systematic review of the literature. The manuscripts describing the toxicities were in print a median of 7.5 years after the relevant drug or device had received initial FDA approval. Subsequent peer-reviewed manuscript publications describing second reports of the toxicities appeared at a median of two years following initial publication. No follow-up reports appeared as peer-reviewed manuscripts for five drugs that had been voluntarily removed from marketing. After FDA approval, 13 Boxed warnings describing the toxicities were included in product labels at a median of 7 years after FDA approval. In six cases, the Boxed warning was issued the same year as the first published report on the ADR, in four cases in the following year, in two cases one year later, in one case three years later. Marketing for six drugs and one device associated with serious toxicities was discontinued, a median of 5 years after FDA approval. Four of these marketing ends happened in the same year as the toxicity manuscript was published, two occurred two years after publication, and one occurred three years after publication.

Clinical scientist leaders for eight pharmaceutical-funded Phase III studies, seeking broadened labels for FDA-approved drugs, unexpectedly reported eight toxicities. These toxicities involved darbepoetin, epoetin, celecoxib, rofecoxib, and valdecoxib. Four phase III clinical trials evaluating epoetin, valdecoxib, and darbepoetin terminated early because of safety concerns. One clinician lead of a safety-focused phase III clinical study for hydroxy-ethyl starch and one lead investigator for an FDA mandated epidemiologic study for phenylpropanolamine (PPA) reported serious toxicities. Five clinician-led case series described six serious toxicities. These side effects were associated with aprotonin, fenfluramine-phentermine, pamidronate, zolendroic acid, levoflxacin, and gadodiamide. One toxicity involving hip replacement prostheses was picked up from an orthopedic surgery registry. Papers reporting follow-up efforts to verify toxicity results were published for 14 toxicities at a median of two years after the first reports of side effects had been published. All but one of these studies confirmed initial very serious ADR findings. The exception was rosiglitazone-associated cardiovascular toxicity.

10.4 Clinical and Economic Impact

Almost 800,000 persons or family members were paid settlements for injuries or deaths resulting from nine toxicities. The weight loss drug, fenfluramine-phentermine, was reported to have injured or led to death for over 600,000 persons. Women with breast cancer or persons with multiple myeloma who developed bisphosphonate-associated osteonecrosis frequently were misdiagnosed by dentists who were not familiar with this syndrome during the years 2000–2003. After several months passed, patients were seen in oral surgery referral practices where debridement was undertaken. After months of treatment, some return of function and reduction in jaw pain occurred. Persons with fenfluramine-phentermine associated cardiac valvulopathy, many of whom were middle-aged women, presented with shortness of breath worsening over weeks to months. Many of the affected women either died or developed cardiac failure. For persons with severe toxicity from epoetin or darbepoetin, presentations included difficult to treat hypertension or cardiac events among persons with chronic kidney disease or venous thromboembolism or tumor progression among cancer patients. Persons with levofloxacin-associated neuropsychiatric toxicity developed agitation or had trouble concentrating, severe muscle and nerve pain, or suicidal thoughts, or, in rare instances, had suicidal attempts. Persons with chronic kidney disease and gadodiamide-associated nephrogenic systemic fibrosis presented with severe fibrosis of the fibrosis and increasingly severe liver, lung, heart, and kidney fibrosis.

10.5 Harms to Clinicians

Eleven of 18 clinicians noted personal or professional harms. Five clinicians reported receiving threats from pharmaceutical manufacturer executives (for rosiglitazone, bisphosphonates, cox-2-inhibitors, and artificial surface replacement hip prostheses). One academic Professor of Medicine lost an academic position after his toxicity report was published. Lawsuits or threats of lawsuits were noted by three physicians. A lead investigator for the phenyl-propanolamine-associated hemorrhagic stroke study, fearing a lawsuit, communicated by telephone only with the FDA. The contract language was interpreted as indicating that a lawsuit would be filed if written communications occurred. One physician who led a Phase III randomized clinical study was sued by a manufacturer for implicating an incorrect product. After filing an error note, the manufacturer dropped the lawsuit. Five physicians who requested permission to present their toxicity findings at FDA advisory committees were refused by FDA coordinator of advisory meetings. This included physicians who had reported toxicities with bisphosphonates, rosiglitazone, and aprotinin. FDA safety personnel noted that the initial adverse event reports for two toxicities (fenfluramine-phentermine-cardiovascular toxicity and bisphosphonate—associated osteonecrosis of the jaw) had been received by the FDA safety division over a period of several months. However, these reports had been included in reports for many other adverse events for the same drugs. They were not easily identified as causing previously unreported cardiac or oral toxicities.

10.6 Harms to Manufacturers, Actions by Regulatory Agencies, Financial Payments, and Attempts to Discredit Physicians

Annual sales for eleven drugs (epoetin, darbepoetin, valdecoxib, celecoxib, rofecoxib rosiglitazone, aprotinin, fenfluramine-phentermine, gadodiamide, phenyl-propanolamine, zolendroic acid, gadodiamide, and hydroxy-ethyl starch) and one device (articular surface replacements) associated with toxicities decreased 94% from $29 billion prior to FDA Advisory Committee meetings to $5 billion following these meetings. Following FDA Advisory Committee meetings, manufacturers stopped marketing of six drugs and one device. Ten manufacturers paid financial settlements for patient injuries (for rosiglitazone, rofecoxib, valdecoxib, celecoxib, fenfluramine-phentermine, epoetin alfa, darbepoetin, hydroxy-ethyl starch, gadodiamide, and articular surface replacement hips). Overall, lawsuit-related payments came to $40 billion. For fenfluramine-phentermine, $22 billion in settlements went to 600,000 claimants. This was the largest payment ever for patient injury. For rofecoxib-associated cardiac toxicities, the manufacturer paid $3.4 billion. The manufacturer of darbepoetin and epoetin paid $615 million in civil settlements and another $160 million in fines. This was the largest payment ever by a biotechnology corporation. For articular surface replacement hip prostheses, the manufacturer paid $4 billion to 8,000 persons for pain, suffering, and hip repair costs.

Manufacturer representatives stated that rosiglitazone, zolendroic acic, pamidronate, epoetin, darbepoetin, articular surface replacement hips, cox-2-inhibitors, fenfluramine-phentermine, gadodiamide, and levofloxacin were unlikely causes of toxicity. A Mayo Clinic and a Fargo Clinic in North Dakota cardiologist together reported the first series of fenfluramine/phentermine-associated cardiac valvulopathies. They had each contacted the manufacturer after diagnosing early cases at their home institutions. Manufacturer employees told each cardiologist that fenfluramine-phentermine was unlikely to be the cause of the valvulopathy.[54] Their collaborative manuscript asserted exactly the opposite. Overall, three manufacturers paid $1.7 billion in fines and settlements for, in part, failing to inform the FDA and clinicians about serious toxicities that occurred with four drugs—valdecoxib ($1.3 billion and $1 billion, respectively), rofecoxib ($321 million and $628 million, respectively), and epoetin and darbepoetin ($150 million and $610 million, respectively).

10.7 Discussion

Very serious ADRs have significant economic, financial, and personal impacts on patients, personal and professional repercussions to physician reporters, and sales and regulatory impacts on manufacturers. In this study, the totality of the ADR impacts represented large human costs in terms of publicly reported payments for safety concerns by manufacturers, public reports of large numbers of injured persons or persons who died from ADRs, large publicly reported clinician costs in terms of loss of job or being involved in litigation with the pharmaceutical manufacturer and large decreases in product sales. While the term "very serious ADRs" is new in the medical literature, prior reports have not systematically evaluated pharmaceuticals or devices that have such large patient, clinical, and manufacturer effects. In interpreting our findings, several factors should be considered.

First, the most common reason for ADR occurrence was class related toxicities identified for three cox-2 inhibitors, two bisphosphonates, and two erythropoiesis stimulating agents. Nine very serious ADRs were caused by six drugs (epoetin, darbepoetin, celecoxib, rofecoxib, valdecoxib, rosiglitazone) that had been evaluated in FDA Phase III licensing trials where no very serious ADRs had emerged. Subsequent Phase III trials identified nine very serious ADRs involving six drugs where study drugs were administered either at higher doses or longer durations than in Phase III licensing trials [4, 5]. Fenfluramine and phentermine are two drugs that were sold to manufacturers by the French pharmaceutical company that manufactured benfluorex, a similar weight loss drug associated with tens of thousands of injured persons.

Second, our findings highlight the importance of Data Safety Monitoring Boards (DSMBs) [3, 6]. Of 20 ADRs evaluated in this report, 40% were first reported to DSMBs evaluating relevant phase III clinical trials. DSMBs for manufacturer-funded clinical trials for valdecoxib, darbepoetin, and epoetin terminated trials early, after cardiovascular toxicity, strokes, and deaths were unexpectedly identified. Rofecoxib toxicity findings led the celecoxib study DSMB chair to pre-emptively convene a cardiovascular adjudication committee [7]. Within six weeks, medical records of patients were reviewed. Although the phase III trial was not terminated early (no safety signal was detected with the sub-study), statistically significant cardiovascular risks were identified at trial end [7]. Phase III studies of valdecoxib, with prospective assessments of cardiovascular events, were terminated by its DSMB when the manufacturer of the related drug, rofecoxib, discontinued marketing [8]. Two co-authors of this study who have been DSMB chairs noted that DSMB members are not indemnified when serving on DSMBs and protocols state that DSMB safety concerns must be reported to study sponsors who in turn report them to the FDA.[SR, OS]. In contrast, three DSMBs included corporate representatives as standing members of the DSMBs. These DSMBs reportedly delayed reporting safety events citing the observation that although deaths were greater with the study drug, investigators did not attribute these deaths to the study drug. As noted by Krumholz, Ross, and Egilman, an important lesson learned from the rofecoxib episode where the DSMB included employees of the sponsoring corporation was that identification of serious ADRs might be delayed if non-independent DSMBs are involved.

Third, while corporate costs of these ADRs were large ($39.8 billion in legal fines and settlements and $24.2 billion in lost revenue), this amount represents probably less than one to two years of sales for the fifteen drugs and one device in our study. Notably, no pharmaceutical executive associated with very serious ADRs paid financial penalties for failing to disclose ADRs.

Fourth, our study identified minimal Institutional Review Board (IRB) involvement in adverse event analyses for zolendroic acid and pamidronate, levofloxacin, fenfluramide-phenteramine, and gadolinium [8, 9] going forward, formal protocols outlining safety focused analyses should be submitted to IRBs. Consideration should be given to forming independent drug safety centers that can assist clinicians with IRB protocol preparation and with interpreting of safety findings. These centers differ in funding, mandate, composition, and function compared with DSMBs, IRBs, FDA Advisory Committees, Steering Committees, and the FDA's Drug Oversight Board, each of whom has formal responsibilities for reviewing drug and device safety.

References

1. Moore TJ, Cohen MR, Furberg CD (2007) Serious adverse drug events reported to the food and drug administration, 1998–2005. Arch Intern Med 167:1752–1759
2. Bennett CL, Schooley B, Taylor M et al (2019) Caveat Medicus: clinician experiences in publishing reports of serious oncology-associated adverse drug reactions. PLoS ONE 14 Article e0219521
3. Rossiter W (2011) A first book of algebra, including the binomial theorem. Nabu Press, Charleston, SC
4. Pfeffer MA, Burdmann EA, Chen C-Y et al (2009)A trial of darbepoetin alfa in type 2 diabetes and chronic kidney disease. N Engl J Med 361:2019–2032
5. Leyland-Jones B, The B.E.S.T. Investigators, Study Group (2003) Breast cancer trial with erythropoietin terminated unexpectedly. Lancet Oncol 4:459–460
6. Singh AK, Szczech L, Tang KL et al (2006) CHOIR investigators. Correction of anemia with epoetin alfa in chronic kidney disease. N Engl J Med 355:2085–2098
7. Solomon SD, McMurray JJ, Pfeffer MA et al (2005) Cardiovascular risk associated with celecoxib in a clinical trial for colorectal adenoma prevention. N Engl J Med 352:1071–1080
8. Nussmeier NA, Whelton AA, Brown MT et al (2005) Complications of the COX-2 inhibitors parecoxib and valdecoxib after cardiac surgery. N Engl J Med 352:1081–1091
9. Connolly HM, Crary JL, McGoon MD et al (1997) Valvular heart disease associated with fenfluramine-phentermine. N Engl J Med 337:581–588

Courtney R. Lubaczewski BA is a graduate of the University of South Carolina Honors College and the co-editor of Cancer Policy with Charles L. Bennett MD Ph.D. MPP. She was a co-author on the 2021 PLOS One article on harms to physicians who report serious adverse drug reactions.

Nancy F. Olivieri MD, MA, MFA, FRCP(C) is a Professor of Pediatrics, Medicine, and Public Health Science at the University of Toronto, Canada. Following training in internal medicine, hematology, and molecular biology, Dr. Olivieri worked in thalassemia, a blood disease primarily of children of emerging countries, for over 30 years, including in Asia through *Hemoglobal*$^{©}$, a charity she founded to improve worldwide care for these children. Over the past 25 years, Dr. Olivieri has been at the center of controversy involving in research integrity, academic freedom, and the protection of patients with thalassemia who were involved in clinical trials funded by industry. Dr. Olivieri teaches a course, *Health and Pharmaceuticals*, to undergraduate and graduate students at the University of Toronto, which explores the influences of the pharmaceutical industry in research and medicine.

William R. Hrushesky MD is an adjunct professor for the University of South Carolina College of Pharmacy and a leading researcher in the area of oncology pharmaceuticals. He was the co-founder of a national company, Oncology Analytics, that is a utilization review provider for the country. He was one of the first clinicians to identify toxicity of erythropoietin. He is a former Professor of Oncology at the University of Minnesota, the State University of New York at Albany, and the University of South Carolina. His prior work on chronobiology included collaborations with Michael Rosbash Ph.D. and Jeffrey Hall Ph.D., the 2017 recipients to the Nobel Prize in Medicine for their discoveries of the molecular mechanisms controlling circadian rhythms. He is an active co-investigator with Dr. Bennett and the SONAR project.

Charles L. Bennett MD, Ph.D. MPP, SmartState Chair and Frank P. and Josie M. Fletcher Chair of Medication Safety and Efficacy and Director, SmartState Center for Medication Safety and Efficacy, is also a Visiting Scholar at the City of Hope National Cancer Institute Designated Comprehensive Cancer Center in Duarte, California and is the co-editor of this book, Cancer

Policy (2nd Edition). Dr. Bennett is a Phi Beta Kappa and High Honors graduate in mathematics from Swarthmore College, earned his medical degree in 1981 from the University of Pennsylvania Perelman School of Medicine, and completed internal medicine, hematology, and oncology training at the Michael Reese Hospital and the University of Chicago Pritzger School of Medicine before completing his Ph.D. and Masters In Public Policy degrees with honors in social science at the RAND Pardee Graduate School of Public Policy in Santa Monica, California. He has led a 20-year National Institutes of Health funded pharmacovigilance called the Research on Adverse Drug events And Reports (RADAR) and subsequently called to Southern Network on Adverse drug Reactions (SONAR) at the University of South Carolina College of Pharmacy.

Moderna, Pfizer-BioNTech, and Johnson & Johnson/Janssen Post-Covid Vaccine Hematological Adverse Events Including Cerebral Venous Sinus Thrombosis (CVST), Thrombotic Thrombocytopenia (VITT), Blood Clots, Increased Vaginal/Menstrual Bleeding and/or Miscarriage, Stillbirth Delivery, or Premature Birth

Oscar Champigneulle and Charles L. Bennett

11.1 Introduction

The Centers for Disease Control (CDC) indicated in 2021 that it would monitor for possible post-COVID-19 vaccination coagulopathy adverse events (AEs). A post-COVID-19 vaccine coagulopathy concern arose over the rare reports of Cerebral Venous Sinus Thrombosis (CVST) with thrombocytopenia and Vaccine-Induced Thromtocytopenic Purpura (VITT) following administration of the Johnson & Johnson/Janssen COVID-19 vaccine.

On April 13, 2021, the CDC and the Food and Drug Administration (FDA) issued a joint statement indicating that they are "reviewing data involving six reported U.S. cases of a rare and severe type of blood clot in individuals after receiving the J&J vaccine. In these cases, a type of blood clot called cerebral venous sinus thrombosis (CVST) was seen in combination with low levels of blood platelets (thrombocytopenia). All six cases occurred among women between the ages of 18 and 48, and symptoms occurred 6–13 days after vaccination."

O. Champigneulle · C. L. Bennett (✉)
SONAR (Southern Network on Adverse Reactions) Program, University of South Carolina College of Pharmacy, Columbia, SC 29208, USA
e-mail: bennettc@cop.sc.edu

O. Champigneulle
e-mail: Oscar_champigneulle@brown.edu

© The Author(s), under exclusive license to Springer Nature Switzerland AG 2022
C. Bennett et al. (eds.), *Cancer Drug Safety and Public Health Policy*,
Cancer Treatment and Research 184, https://doi.org/10.1007/978-3-031-04402-1_11

It is reported that "six women, ages 18–48, developed rare cerebral venous sinus thrombosis, which are blood clots in combination with low levels of blood platelets. One of the recipients died, and another is in critical condition." Based on these six reported cases, the CDC and FDA recommended a pause in the delivery of J&J vaccine.

On April 14, 2021, the CDC Advisory Committee on Immunization Practice s (ACIP) held a hearing to address Johnson & Johnson/Janssen vaccine CVST with thrombocytopenia and VITT concerns. At this meeting, the ACIP decided to continue the pause on providing Johnson & Johnson/Janssen COVID-19 vaccine until additional data are available, including data related to thrombopenia without CVST and data on VITT cases.

On April 23, 2021, the CDC lifted the pause on the J&J vaccine.

11.1.1 Study Implementation

Our study, started February 17, 2021, includes review of thrombocytopenia and other blood clot related AEs reported to the CDC Vaccine Adverse Event Reporting System (VAERS) and a second set of similar cases identified in social media. This study was implemented, in part, because we recognized that social media serves as a platform for individuals to share opinions and experiences with the general public related to a wide range of topics, including healthcare. We wanted to determine (1) if, with the onset of the pandemic and the recent release of three COVID-19 vaccines, including the Johnson & Johnson (J&J) vaccine, individuals have taken to discussing COVID-19 and vaccines in a virtual environment and (2) are there similar cases reported to the CDC's VAERs, the nationally recognized vaccine adverse event reporting system database? Specifically, this study examined if individuals were (1) sharing COVID-19 adverse event experiences related to hemorrhagic complications on social media and (2) were reporting VITT, CVST, thrombotic, and hemorrhagic complications to the CDC VAERS. These four outcomes were selected as the foci of this pilot study as they are clinical events that are recognizable to persons who have been vaccinated, some of whom may not visit a physician or pharmacist for evaluation (and hence will end up only on social media sites). The overall aim of this pilot study is to investigate if joint use of social media and VAERS might identify a subset of severe life-threatening COVID-19 vaccine related AEs that would not have been immediately evident from VAERS analyses only.

11.2 Methods

From February 17, 2021 through April 13, 2021, the social media platform, Twitter, was searched to identify individuals claiming to have experienced possible previously unrecognized or under-recognized thrombotic or hemorrhagic side effects following COVID-19 vaccination. We began the search looking for event such as blood clots, petechiae, bruising, bleeding in the mouth or gums, or blood in urine, vomit, or stool. Twitter key words included "Covid vaccine side effects," "Covid vaccine petechiae side effects," "Covid vaccine bleeding side effects," "Covid vaccine blood clots," "Covid vaccine thrombopenia," and the like. As a result of this search, it was discovered that several COVID-19 vaccine recipients reportedly experienced various findings including vaginal/menstrual bleeding-related adverse events shortly after receiving COVID-19 vaccinations. We then searched Twitter specifically using the key words "Covid vaccine menstrual side effects," "COVID-19 vaccine period side effects," "COVID-19 vaccine vaginal side effects," and so forth. As a result of this search, it was discovered that some of these individuals reported experiencing miscarriages after COVID-19 vaccination so further searches were conducted specifically related to "Covid vaccine pregnancy" and "Covid vaccine miscarriage."

Once potential COVID-19 vaccine thrombotic and hemorrhagic side effects were identified, the CDC Vaccine AEs System (VAERS) was searched to determine if there were cases reported in the CDC database related to the potential AEs we had identified on Twitter: thrombosis, thrombocytopenia, blood clots, hemorrhage, vaginal/menstrual bleeding, and miscarriage.

Based on the April 13, 2021 CDC and FDA stated concerns about CVST in combination with thrombocytopenia, Twitter was searched to determine if there were discussions related to these concerns. VAERS was then searched to determine if there were AEs related to CVST, VITT, thrombocytopenia, or other blood clotting related AEs.

11.3 Results

On Twitter, 21 posts were identified pertaining to thrombosis or hemorrhage. In the CDC VAERS database containing post-COVID-19 vaccination AEs, we identified the following AEs, some of which were reported for each of the three COVID-19 vaccines:

- 340 cases of thrombocytopenia and/or blood clotting related AEs
- 85 cases of vaginal/menstrual bleeding related AEs (including increases in bleeding, abnormal time frame for cycles, excessive cramping, and early onset of bleeding)
- 98 cases of miscarriage, stillbirth delivery, or premature birth cases.

These individuals had received at least one dose of the Moderna, Pfizer-BioNTech, or Johnson & Johnson/Janssen COVID-19 vaccines and reported blood clots related issues, vaginal/menstrual bleeding, and/or miscarriage, stillbirth delivery, premature birth, or thrombocytopenia-related AEs starting within days of receiving a first or second dose of vaccine.

Although the CDC and FDA have expressed concern about the blood clot related AE CVST with thrombocytopenia, related to the J&J vaccine, this study found blood clot related AEs, not including CVST with thrombocytopenia, reported related to all three COVID-19 vaccines: Moderna, Pfizer-BioNTech, and J&J.

We tracked VAERS data COVID-19 vaccine AEs weekly following our initial review. As of May 7, 2021, we identified the following:

VAERS COVID-19 vaccine adverse events as of May 7, 2021

	Moderna	Pfizer	J&J	Total
Vaginal/Menstrual Bleeding related AEs	45	51	75	171
Miscarriage, stillbirth delivery, or premature birth related AEs	40	81	19	140
Clotting related AEs	401	551	620	1572
Bleeding, other hematological AEs	768	841	439	2048
Total	1254	1524	1153	3931

11.3.1 Blood Clot Related Events

From February 17, 2021 through April 13, 2021, this study identified no one discussing post-COVID-19 vaccine blood clot related issues on Twitter. However, given that on April 13, 2021 the CDC and FDA paused the use of the J&J vaccine for blood clot related issues, the VAERS data base was searched for the following terms relating to VITT or CVST and thrombocytopenia: bleeding, bleed, thrombocytopenia, thrombosis, thrombus, blood clot, platelet, cerebral venous thrombosis, CVST, VITT, cerebral venous thrombocytopenia, and deep vein thrombosis. The search identified the following recurring AEs reported to VAERS: thrombocytopenia, thrombopenia, nosebleed, bleeding gums, bleeding eyes, bleeding ears, internal bleeding, petechiae, excessive bleeding from a cut, blood clot, clot, thrombosis, thrombus, immune thrombocytopenia purpura, gastrointestinal bleeding, low platelet count, blood in urine, blood in stool, and rectal bleeding.

The VAERS search identified 401 Moderna blood clot related adverse event cases, 551 Pfizer BioNTech cases, and 620 J&J cases for a total of 1,572 VAERS blood clot related events. As noted by the CDC, VAERS reports do not infer causal relationships.

The chart below highlights some of the most significant reports.

Additional examples of VAERS blood clot related reports are included in Table 11.1. Individuals who had received at least one dose of the Moderna, Pfizer-BioNTech, or J&J COVID-19 vaccines and reported adverse events (AEs) starting within days of vaccination.

Table 11.1 Examples of COVID-19 vaccine AE reports

Drug Maker	Date vaccinated	# Doses	Gender	Event date	Age
Moderna	12/4/20	Unknown	female	1/12/21	33 years old
#Right parietal/temporal subarachnoid hemorrhage and right intra-axial hemorrhage CT brain (1/12/21): Right parietal intra-axial hemorrhage toward the convexity measuring 2.3 × 1.1 × 1.7 cm with decompression into the subarachnoid space, mild right predominantly temporal and parietal subarachnoid hemorrhage is seen with minimal associated hemorrhage along the tentorium. Mild diffuse right cerebral sulcal effacement with minimal leftward midline shift measuring 2.5 mm. #Dural sinus thrombosis CTA head (1/11/21): Increased density within the superior sagittal sinus, inferior sagittal sinus, and transverse sinuses on noncontrasted images with no flow seen on postcontrast sequences consistent with venous sinus thrombosis #Left sided weakness 2/2 above #Recent jaw alignment procedure					
Pfizer-BioNTech	1/4/21	1	male	1/11/21	80 years old
"80YO male who htn, cva, epilepsy, ckd, cerebral avm s/p repair, cad s/p cab, cva (left sided hemiplegia) , hx of prostate cancer recent admission for pna on abx presents to ED on 1/11 with dizziness, hypoxia. CT with Bilateral PE" "Large bilateral pulmonary artery emboli in the right and left main pulmonary artery extending into the right and left main pulmonary artery branches bilaterally. Findings are associated with right-sided heart strain." "Patchy alveolar airspace disease within the lungs highly suspicious for COVID pneumonia" "Covid negative. Patients wife recovered from COVID-19 infection within last month. Patent thus far has tested negative. Doppler lower extremity revealed Acute occlusive vein thrombosis of the entire course of the gastrocnemius vein and soleal vein. Patient received covid vaccine on 1/4/21. Patient has several risk factors for clot—age, previous CVA, hx of prostate cancer. Also had positive covid exposure though tested negative"					
J&J	3/6/21	1	female	3/12/21	35 years old
Diagnosis: Cortical vein thrombosis, massive intracerebral hemorrhage with tentorial herniation, thrombocytopenia. Clinical Presentation and Course: 1 week after receiving Janssen COVID19 vaccination, patient developed gradually worsening headache. On March 17th, patient presented to Hospital with dry heaving, sudden worsening of headache and L sided weakness. Evaluation with head CT revealed a large R temporoparietal intraparenchymal hemorrhage with 1.3cm midline shift. She ended up getting intubated for worsening mental status. On evaluation at arrival in Medical Center, she was noted to have extensor posturing. Repeat imaging revealed worsening midline shift to 1.6cm. CTA showed cortical vein thrombosis involving the right transverse and sigmoid sigmoid sinus with tentorial herniation. Patient developed brain herniation and brain death was pronounced on March 18th, 2021.					
Moderna	1/27/21	1	Female	1/29/21	30 years old
Central venous sinus thrombosis					

(continued)

Table 11.1 (continued)

Drug Maker	Date vaccinated	# Doses	Gender	Event date	Age
Pfizer-BioNTech	2/17/21	Unknown	Male	2/20/21	85 years old
THROMBOTIC STROKE IN THE DISTRIBUTION OF THE LEFT MCA DISTRIBUTION					
Pfizer-BioNTech	1/30/21	2	Female	1/31/21	87 years old
right middle cerebral stroke due to clot in brain; right middle cerebral stroke due to clot in brain; This is a spontaneous report from a contactable consumer or other non hcp. A 87-year-old female patient received the second dose of BNT162B2 (PFIZER-BIONTECH COVID-19 VACCINE, lot# EL9265), via an unspecified route of administration right arm single dose on 30Jan2021 15:00 for COVID-19 immunisation. First dose was received on 09Jan2021 03:00 PM, right arm, lot # EK9231. Medical history included diabetes mellitus, hypertension, hyperthyroidism, glaucoma, drug allergy (to Sulfites). The patient's concomitant medications were not reported. The patient experienced right middle cerebral stroke due to clot in brain from 31 Jan 2021. The patient was hospitalized from 31 Jan 2021 to 01 Feb 2021. The events outcome was not recovered.					
Moderna	2/19/21	2	Male	3/7/21	90 years old
Death on March 8 due to a large blood clot at the base of his brain. This was 16 days after innoculation					
Pfizer-BioNTech	2/1/21	Unknown	Female	2/1/21	83 years old
My mother called me when she was going to get her second vaccination. She was alive and well and living independently at her home. She could walk, talk, make her own food, wash and dry her own clothes and take her own baths. After taking the second vaccination she went downhill. She became sicker and sicker and eventually she started coughing up blood. She decided to go to the hospital, another Hospital of facility. I don't know what the treatment was at that hospital but she was soon transferred to facility and that is where I was notified she was in the hospital and visited her there. After arriving they intubated her and said she had blood clots in her brain and heart. When I saw her after she transferred from Hospital to the Hospital I noticed one arm was swollen. Her legs were as they have been for the last 20 years and looked okay to me–no discoloration other than her regular discoloring at one right ankle and the same old same old slight swelling in the left ankle. The doctors and nurses were putting the blame on her legs but you could tell things were happening elsewhere. But as she got worse and worse at the hospital her right arm become more and more swollen with dark bruises appearing–the hospital staff took pictures. The left arm continued to swell and did not look normal at all. She apparently had bleeding in her left lung from a blood clot. She had three areas of her brain that add clots and some bleeding. She was constipated and gaseous when they cleaned her. They didn't treat her constipation which made being intubated worse because I feel that caused her intestines to swell, thus she also had bleeding in her intestines. My mother died on March 17, 2021 at hospital in ICU. I was told they could not treat the blood clots because of the bleeding in her lung, intestines and brain.					
J&J	3/8/21	1	female	3/17/21	38 years old
The patient was experiencing headaches 1 week ago. She also had aphasia later in the week. She went to an outside hospital on 3/24/2021 and was found to have intraparenchymal hemorrhage in addition to venous sinus thrombosis. She is being treated for the venous sinus thrombosis with heparin					

11.3.2 Vaginal/Menstrual Bleeding AEs

From February 17, 2021 through April 13, 2021, this study identified 15 cases of vaginal/menstrual-related post-COVID-19 vaccination AEs posted by women on Twitter. These individuals, who had received at least one dose of the COVID-19 vaccine, claimed to have experienced at least one of the following: onset of vaginal/menstrual bleeding during the overall height of the post-vaccine adverse effects experienced; extended vaginal/menstrual bleeding, sometimes continuing for more than 2 weeks; and irregular vaginal/menstrual cycles, including premature spotting. Several of these women referenced more than 40 other individuals who reportedly experienced similar post-COVID-19 symptoms. The following chart highlights some of the specific comments posted on Twitter by these women.

After finding the menstrual related posts on Twitter, the CDC VAERS database was searched for AEs related to vaginal/menstrual bleeding.

In the CDC VAERS database containing more than 50,000 post-COVID-19 vaccination AEs, we identified 85 cases of vaginal/menstrual bleeding related AEs (including increases in bleeding, abnormal time frame for cycles, excessive cramping, and early onset of bleeding).

Examples of VAERS vaginal/menstrual bleeding related reports included in Table 11.2. These individuals had received at least one dose of the Moderna, Pfizer-BioNTech, or J&J COVID-19 vaccines and reported AEs starting within days of vaccination. As noted by the CDC, VAERS reports do not infer causal relationships.

Table 11.2 Examples of comments posted on Twitter about vaginal/menstrual bleeding related COVID-19 vaccine AEs

"The new COVID side effect is dysmenorrhea and people are having 15 day long periods"
"I have seen more than 40 women report on a social media group that after the (Pfizer) COVID-19 vaccine they had unusual spotting followed by early menses. It (also) happened to my wife"
"After my first dose my menses = super unusual. I wondered if it had something to do with the vaccine."
"I had the slightest spotting, no cramps but pain that I usually got when I had periods. Mind you, my periods stopped over a year ago."
"I personally heard of people bleed after the vaccine (Pfizer and Moderna). Your period might start early or you might get menstrual pain without any bleeding. I personally got the last one."
"If you experienced menstrual irregularities as a side symptom of Covid-you may also experience them with the vaccine. I've had my second dose and the same period problems I had when sick."
"Several friends I know in the healthcare profession have stated that the Covid Vaccine has made some women experience longer than usual menstrual cycles that are heavy from start to finish."

Table 11.3 Examples of comments posted on Twitter about miscarriage related COVID-19 vaccine AEs

Sara Beltrán Ponce MD was 14 weeks pregnant when she misguidedly volunteered to get a "2nd dose of Pfizer's mRNA Covid "vaccine" despite numerous warnings of safety concerns for pregnant women and their unborn babies. 6 days later she had a miscarriage"
"This year I changed jobs, moved interstate into a covid hotspot, lost weight, got pregnant, and miscarried after getting vaccine"
"My official statements to my pregnant patients or those considering pregnancy & wondering if to get the mRNA vaccines? Make an informed choice but strongly consider getting it. Risk of COVID-19 disease includes miscarriage, preterm birth, heart attack, prolonged hospitalization"
"People need to look the covid vaccine data coming out of USA. How many women suffered miscarriages after having the vax"

11.3.3 Miscarriage, Stillbirth Delivery, or Premature Birth AEs

From February 17, 2021 through April 13, 2021, this study identified six cases of miscarriage post-COVID-19 vaccination AEs posted on Twitter. The following table highlights some of the specific comments posted on Twitter relate to miscarriage.

After finding the COVID-19 vaccine miscarriage related posts on Twitter, the CDC VAERS database was searched for AEs related to miscarriage, stillbirth delivery, or premature birth. In the CDC VAERS database containing more than 50,000 post-COVID-19 vaccination AEs, we identified 98 cases of miscarriage, stillbirth delivery, or premature birth.

Examples of VAERS miscarriage, stillbirth delivery, or premature birth reports are included in Table 11.3. As noted by the CDC, VAERS reports do not infer causal relationships.

Johnson and Johnson/Janssen reports of CVST include the one case that appears to be one of the six cases that the ACIP reviewed yesterday.

11.4 Conclusions

Reports of blood clot related AEs were reported to VAERS and/or were identified in social media related to three COVID-19 vaccines used in the United States: Moderna, Pfizer-BioNTech, and J&J. There were also been reports of blood clot related adverse events after administration of the AstraZeneca COVID-19 vaccine used outside the United States. Reports of CVST with thrombocytopenia were associated with the J&J and the AstraZeneca vaccines.

Through Twitter posts, we identified two signals of potential novel post-COVID-19 vaccine associated AEs, primarily gender-specific: (1) vaginal/menstrual bleeding and (2) miscarriage, stillbirth delivery, or premature birth. Additionally, the CDC and FDA identified CVST in combination with thrombocytopenia as a concern related to the J&J vaccine.

Although the VAERS data identified 171 reports of vaginal/menstrual bleeding adverse events, 140 reports of miscarriage, stillbirth delivery, or premature birth, 1,572 reports of clotting-related adverse events, and 2,048 reports of other hematological adverse events following COVID-19 vaccination, the numbers of these possible adverse event reports for these toxicities may be significantly higher, given that a It should be noted that a 2010 Harvard Pilgrim Health Plan grant report, "Electronic Support for Public Health–Vaccine Adverse Event Reporting System (ESP:VAERS)" found that "fewer than 1% of vaccine adverse events are reported." This means that the actual number of COVID-19 vaccine adverse events may be as high as 17,100 for vaginal/menstrual bleeding AEs, as high as 14,000 adverse events related to miscarriage, stillbirth delivery, or premature birth, as high as 157,200 reports of clotting-related AEs, and as high as 204,800 other hematological-related AEs.

Clearly, as with all adverse event evaluations, our data do not infer causal relationships. Ongoing research is need regarding whether COVID-19 vaccination is strongly associated with blood clot related concerns, vaginal bleeding, and/or miscarriages, stillbirth delivery, or premature birth and, if so, investigation of potential causal routes, particularly antibodies for CVST and VITT, is required.

Our study suggests that social media platforms, like Twitter, may provide a new source of adverse event identification following COVID-19 vaccination. Following such identification, the VAERS database should be searched to determine if such potential AEs are being reported to the CDC. The authors of this study support COVID-19 vaccination but encourage acknowledgement and investigation of the full continuum of potential vaccine AEs.

Oscar Champigneulle is a junior at Brown University in Providence, Rhode Island. During a semester that was interrupted by absence of in-person classes due to the COVID-19 pandemic, he conducted investigations of pharmaceutical safety. His two foci were hematologic complications of COVID-19 vaccinations and disability-related complications following fluroquinolone administration.

Charles L. Bennett MD, Ph.D., MPP, SmartState Chair and Frank P. and Josie M. Fletcher Chair of Medication Safety and Efficacy and Director, SmartState Center for Medication Safety and Efficacy, is also a Visiting Scholar at the City of Hope National Cancer Institute Designated Comprehensive Cancer Center in Duarte, California and is the co-editor of this book, Cancer Policy (2nd Edition). Dr. Bennett is a Phi Beta Kappa and High Honors graduate in mathematics from Swarthmore College, earned his medical degree in 1981 from the University of Pennsylvania Perelman School of Medicine, and completed internal medicine, hematology, and oncology training at the Michael Reese Hospital and the University of Chicago Pritzger School of Medicine before completing his Ph.D. and Masters In Public Policy degrees with honors in social science at the RAND Pardee Graduate School of Public Policy in Santa Monica, California. He has led a 20-year National Institutes of Health funded pharmacovigilance called the Research on Adverse Drug events And Reports (RADAR) and subsequently called to Southern Network on Adverse drug Reactions (SONAR) at the University of South Carolina College of Pharmacy.

Investigating Novel Genetic Markers for Fluoroquinolone Associated Disorders

Andrew Bennett

12.1 Introduction

Fluoroquinolones (FQs) are among the most commonly prescribed class of antibiotics and have regulatory approval to treat anthrax, pneumonia, unitary tract infections, and sinus infection among other uses. The three main FQs are Cipro-floxacin, Levofloxacin, and Moxifloxacin. In 2017, over 22 million prescriptions of these FQs were dispensed in the United States. Despite their popularity, many patients appeared to have experienced severe adverse reactions that were not previously noted as being associated with FQ use. One serious toxicity, Fluoroquinolone Associated Disability (FQAD), was identified by the Food and Drug Administration and by a large number of FQ-treated persons [1]. FQAD is characterized by disability of 12 months or longer and toxicity affecting two or more organ systems (frequently FQAD is associated with neuropsychiatric toxicity). Patients with FQAD came together as a social network seeking to partner with scientists who would investigate causes of FQAD and possible treatments. Through collaboration of this network with researchers at the University of South Carolina, whole-exome sequencing of DNA obtained from sputum samples of 25 persons with FQAD was performed [2]. Several possible genetic markers that may predispose patients to FQ-associated neuropsychiatric toxicity were identified. One genetic marker is the CYP2D6 gene. Of the initial 25 patients, 13 (56.52%) expressed mutations in CYP2D6. Of the thirteen individuals with this genetic marker, ten had significant cognitive impairment. A follow-up study has received IRB approval and will investigate the prevalence of CYP2D6 mutations in a second sample of 100 persons with FQ-associated neuropsychiatric toxicity, as well as seek to identify other potential genetic markers [3].

A. Bennett (✉)
SONAR (Southern Network on Adverse Reactions) Program, University of South Carolina College of Pharmacy, Columbia, SC 29208, USA
e-mail: andrew.bennett@pharm.ox.ac.uk

© The Author(s), under exclusive license to Springer Nature Switzerland AG 2022
C. Bennett et al. (eds.), *Cancer Drug Safety and Public Health Policy*,
Cancer Treatment and Research 184, https://doi.org/10.1007/978-3-031-04402-1_12

12.1.1 Timeline of Events

2011

Persons with FQ-associated neuropsychiatric toxicity created a social network that they termed the FLOXed Network. Three FQs, ciprofloxacin, moxifloxacin, and levofloxacin, are commonly prescribed antibiotics that are approved by the Food and Drug Administration (FDA) for treatment of urinary tract infections, sinus infections, and pneumonia. These individuals with FQ-associated neuropsychiatric toxicity as a group felt that their medical concerns were not being adequately evaluated by their physicians. Following a chance encounter at a FDA meeting on patients and adverse drug reactions with one of the FLOXed members and Charles L Bennett MD Ph.D. MPP, the leadership of the FLOXed Network began to collaborate with the Southern Network on Adverse Reactions (SONAR), National Institutes of Health R01 funded drug safety network (Dr. Bennett is the principal investigator for SONAR) seeking to collaboratively investigate the causes and treatments of FQAD. This marks the beginning of the grassroots movement that would prove vital in providing persons with FQAD opportunities to participate in research studies.

2014

The FLOXed Network and SONAR collaborated to petition the FDA seeking to require FQ manufacturers to revise the product labels to be more informative about FQ-associated toxicities. Citizen petitions represent a process that is open to any citizen in the United States allowing individuals to communicate with Federal agencies such as the FDA and engage in a dialogue. Citizen Petitions with the FDA generally request that the FDA require manufacturers of certain pharmaceuticals to affect some change, typically in the form of adding a warning in the FDA-approved package insert. The first citizen petition request was to add to the package insert a statement that the mechanism of action of FQAD was directly related to mitochondrial toxicity. This claim was denied in 2015 [4]. The second citizen petition was to add a warning to the package insert of FQs that warned of potential neuropsychiatric adverse events. This would ultimately be accepted, but not for four years [5].

2015

FDA epidemiologist Debra Boxwell presents in a meeting with an FDA Advisory Committee meeting to evaluate the potential risks and benefits of FQs [1]. Here, the term FQAD is formally defined as a range of disabling symptoms that significantly inhibit or disrupt a person's ability to conduct normal life functions with the caveat that the symptoms must persist for at least 30 days. The symptoms must involve two or more of the following organ systems: musculoskeletal, neuropsychiatric, peripheral nervous system, sensory (sight, sound, etc....) skin, and/or cardiovascular. The FDA Advisory Committee voted 20–1 in favor of Boxwell, i.e. confirming FQAD as a new and serious toxicity of FQ antibiotics [3].

FDA notifies SONAR that the Citizen Petition related to FQs and mitochondrial toxicity has been denied [4].

2016

A study conducted by SONAR project injected mice with Ciprofloxacin to investigate what toxicities might arise [6]. In this study, five groups of mice received Ciprofloxacin with increments of 10 mg per kg of mouse. The first group started at 10 mg/kg and a sixth control group received no Ciprofloxacin. The treated mice were found to have lower grip strengths, reduced balance, and depressive behavior when compared with the control group. Beyond the mice, the study also included a survey to the patients of the FQAD network conducted by SONAR and the FLOXed Network. Of 94 persons with FQ-associated toxicities who responded, 93 were found to experience adverse neuropsychiatric events such as anxiety, depression, clouded thinking, and suicidal ideation. Furthermore, several respondents reported to have taken only one dose of Ciprofloxacin and experienced these symptoms within days of taking the drug [6]. Ultimately, this study was important because it showed that the affected mice were having similar toxicities to the FQAD patients.

2017

The findings of the first phase of the genetic study to investigate the genetic markers for FQAD were presented at a VA conference for hematologists and oncologists [2]. The objective of this study was to identify which genes could be responsible for FQAD. Mutations in these genes would thus be genetic markers that could be used to identify patients who are at higher risk of FQAD. Saliva was collected from 25 of these patients, and whole exome sequencing was performed on the samples. The study consisted of 24 individuals who were predominately white (82.61%), female (65.22%), and under the age of 40 (61%). The remaining saliva sample was not used for this study. Importantly, 16 of the 24 had genetic mutations to the CYP2D6 gene. A genetic marker had thus been identified. The patients with the genetic marker had been prescribed FQs for urinary tract infections more than any other ailment. Also, eight of those with the genetic marker had severe gastrointestinal distress, three had persistent headaches, and ten experienced severe cognitive impairment. Besides CYP2D6, the whole exome sequencing of the 24 patients revealed that there were likely other genetic mutations that were overrepresented FQAD. Each other possible candidate was in some way related to the Cytochrome P450 class of proteins.

2018

The FDA responds to the second citizen petition from 2014, and the black box warnings are upgraded to include neuropsychiatric toxicity as a potential AE [5].

2019

A second genetic study begins and again reaches out to the social network group. Within the first day, hundreds of patients suffering from FQAD sent emails to the study investigators requesting to be included in the second study.

2021

After six months of review, the University of South Carolina Institutional Research Board (IRB) grants approval for the study to gather saliva samples from 100 patients as well as collect relevant information through a detailed survey.

12.1.2 Background of CYP2D6

It is necessary to understand the relationship between CYP2D6 genes and FQs to explain why identifying genetic markers is critical in identifying at-risk patients [7]. The "CYP" root in CYP2D6 stands for Cytochrome P450, so CYP2D6 then describes all the nucleotides that make up one of the many genes that will be transcribed and then translated into the Cytochrome P450 proteins. The 450 refers to the wavelength at which the absorption of incoming photons is at its maximum. CYP2D6 is just one of many genes that make up the CYP family of genes. The P450 proteins are found in virtually all organisms, signifying their importance to complex life. They contribute to carbon source assimilation, biosynthesis of hormones, and most relevant to FQ, degradation of xenobiotics [8]. Xenobiotics are, in short, substances that are not native to the host organism [8]. A common example of xenobiotics are pharmaceuticals, of which FQs are indeed one. Because P450 proteins are involved in the breakdown of organic molecules, they are classified as enzymes. CYP2D6 is one of the most important genes for the creation of enzymes that break down pharmaceuticals. In fact, up to a quarter of all known drugs are metabolized by the proteins created by CYP2D6. CYP2D6 also is highly polymorphic, which means there exists in the population many mutations to the gene that alter the function of the resulting proteins. When an enzyme is altered, it often loses its ability to metabolize its substrates as efficiently, and P450 enzymes are no different [6]. Since CYP2D6 creates enzymes that break down drugs in the liver, which is also where FQs are metabolized, it was likely (based on the initial whole exome sequencing results) that the high number of polymorphisms in the CYP2D6 were the culprit for the resulting FQAD [2].

One study conducted by Marez et al. in 1997 aimed to investigate the phenotypic results of several polymorphisms for the CYP2D6 gene [9]. Marez's study described 48 point mutations, of which 29 were completely new phenotypic expressions. Over half of the resulting mutations were 1749 G$\rightarrow$C, 2938 C$\rightarrow$T, and 4268 G$\rightarrow$C mutations. These point mutations were found to result in a significant decrease in the ability of P450 enzymes to metabolize drugs. All the mutations observed were located in the intron–exon boundaries, which means that they are located near the end of the coding regions of the genes [9]. The results of this study highlight how precarious the CYP2D6 genes are. A single point mutation could result in a catastrophic inability to metabolize drugs.

12.2 Conclusion

A common sentiment these patients share is not one of anger or frustration, but one of concern for future recipients of FQs. Many want closure for what has been a life-long consequence of taking an antibiotic, sometimes only for one dose. Black box updates and FDA recognition of FQAD has been small victories for the FQ patients, but the end goal of all this is to prevent further FQADs. Identification of genetic markers serves as one step toward this goal, and this can only be done through the ongoing cooperation with FQAD patients.

References

1. FDA Briefing Document - Joint Meeting of the Antimicrobial Drugs Advisory Committee and the Drug Safety and Risk Management Advisory Committee (2015). The benefits and risks of systemic fluoroquinolone antibacterial drugs for the treatment of Acute Bacterial Sinusitis (ABS), Acute Bacterial Exacerbation of Chronic Bronchitis in Patients Who Have Chronic Obstructive Pulmonary Disease (ABECB-COPD), and uncomplicated urinary tract infections (uUTI). https://www.fda.gov/downloads/advisorycommittees/committeesmeetingmaterials/drugs/anti-infectivedrugsadvisorycommittee/ucm467383.pdf. Accessed 51 May /2021
2. Bennett A, Qureshi ZP, Bennett CL (2017) A novel genetic marker has been identified in patients with FQ-associated neuropsychatric toxicity. Conference proceedings for the Association of veterans administration hematologist and oncologist. (abstract 55). https://www.mdedge.com/fedprac/avaho/article/146822/novel-genetic-marker-has-been-identified-patients-fluoroquinolone. Accessed 1 May 2021
3. Marchant J (2018) When antibiotics turn toxic. Nature 555:431–433
4. Woodcock J (2015) FDA. Denial response from FDA to the Southern Network on Adverse Reactions (SONAR) regarding levaquin and mitochrondrial toxicity. https://www.regulations.gov/document?D=FDA-2014-P-1505-0005. Accessed 1 May 2021
5. Woodcock J (2018) FDA. Partial approval and partial denial response from FDA to the Southern Network on Adverse Reactions (SONAR) regarding levaquin. https://www.regulations.gov/document?D=FDA-2014-P-1611-0005. Accessed 1 May 2021
6. Kaur K, Fayad R, Saxena A, Frizzell N, Chanda A, Das S, The Southern Network on Adverse Reactions (SONAR) project (2016) Fluoroquinolone-related neuropsychiatric and mitochondrial toxicity: a collaborative investigation by scientists and members of a social network. J Commun Support Oncol 14(2):54–65. https://doi.org/10.12788/jcso.0167
7. Werck-Reichhart D, Feyereisen R (2021) Cytochromes P450: a success story. Genome Biol 2000. https://genomebiology.biomedcentral.com/articles, https://doi.org/10.1186/gb-2000-1-6-reviews3003. Accessed 1 May 2021

8. Lu K, Mahbub, Ridwan, Fox, James G (2018) Xenobiotics: interaction with the intestinal microflora. ILAR J 56:218–227
9. Marez D, Legrand M, Sabbagh N et al (1997) Polymorphism of the cytochrome P450 CYP2D6 gene in a European population: characterization of 48 mutations and 53 alleles, their frequencies and evolution. Pharmacogenetics 7:193–202

Andrew Bennett BA is a graduate of the University of South Carolina Honors Program with a Magna Cum Laude award. He was funded in part by grants from the American Cancer Society Institutional Research Grant Award and the University of South Carolina's Science Undergraduate Research Fellowship under the leadership of Zaina Qureshi, Ph.D. and Carolyn Bannister, Ph.D. to investigate genetic risk factors for fluoroquinolone-associated disability. The initial work was presented in 2017 at the Association of Veteran's Administration Hematology and Oncology conference in Denver and covered in more detail in Nature in a news article by Jo Marchant "When antibiotics turn toxic: commonly prescribed drugs called fluoroquinolones cause rare, disturbing side effects. Researchers are struggling to work out why." (March 7, 2018; 555: 431–438). He will begin post-graduate studies focusing on quinolone-associated toxicity at Oxford University in England in October 2021.

Index